"This book is an important tool for educators and therapists to help children with ASD learn to think 'inside the box.' Rehearsing social situations is key to anxiety reduction and peer acceptance in teenagers who simply don't know what to do or say in a variety of common situations.

This book is a 'must have' for parents. Instead of the author simply teaching the child how to respond in a situation, this book uses discussion questions to help parents teach children their own preferred responses to situations. This helps the parents tailor the strategies to reflect each family's unique beliefs."

—*Joann Pesavento, Behavioral Specialist Consultant specializing in children with Autism Spectrum Disorders*

"Lisa Timms' *60 Social Situations* is a great resource for therapists, guidance counselors and parents alike. It helps break down a variety of socially-related scenarios that are often complicated and confusing for teenagers on the autism spectrum. The questions that accompany each topic are thought provoking and applicable to everyday life and generalize easily into the real world. It also provides parents with a stepping stone to generate very important discussions with their teens with experiences they may have already had or are likely to have."

—*Deanne Chincola, Clinical Supervisor in Behavioral Health Rehabilitation Services*

"Finally, a useful and relevant guide about appropriate and safe social interactions has emerged that can really help teens and young adults with an Autism Spectrum Disorder. Lisa Timms has written a top-notch book that includes skills development scenarios for school, recreation, community, social networking, and employment. Information for parents to coach and facilitate skills is positive, helpful, and thought provoking. *60 Social Situations and Discussion Starters* is easy to read, fun to discuss, and a great book to improve the understanding of social situations."

—*Donna Podrazik, Psy.D., Licensed Psychologist, Private Practice*

"This is an invaluable tool to aid in the improvement of social skills. I have been waiting for something like this! It has the potential to diminish or limit the negative consequences, i.e. anxiety, depression and loss of self esteem, that often accompany a poor social skill set. I highly recommend it to parents of ASD and typical teens. In our home we would pick a topic and discuss it at the dinner table. I know it will give parents a sense of peace of mind, that they might better prepare their teen for the unknown."

—*Mary Walsh, parent*

of related interest

The Complete Guide to Asperger's Syndrome
Tony Attwood
ISBN 978 1 84310 495 7 (hardback)
ISBN 978 1 84310 669 2 (paperback)

Freaks, Geeks and Asperger Syndrome
A User Guide to Adolescence
Luke Jackson
Foreword by Tony Attwood
ISBN 978 1 84310 098 0

The Social and Life Skills MeNu
A Skill Building Workbook for Adolescents with Autism Spectrum Disorders
Karra M. Barber
ISBN 978 1 84905 861 2

The ASD Workbook
Understanding Your Autism Spectrum Disorder
Penny Kershaw
ISBN 978 1 84905 195 8

Social Skills for Teenagers and Adults with Asperger Syndrome
A Practical Guide to Day-to-Day Life
Nancy J. Patrick
ISBN 978 1 84310 876 4

60 SOCIAL SITUATIONS & DISCUSSION STARTERS to Help Teens on the Autism Spectrum Deal with Friendships, Feelings, Conflict and More

SEEING THE BIG PICTURE

LISA A. TIMMS

Jessica Kingsley *Publishers*
London and Philadelphia

First published in 2011
by Jessica Kingsley Publishers
116 Pentonville Road
London N1 9JB, UK
and
400 Market Street, Suite 400
Philadelphia, PA 19106, USA

www.jkp.com

Library of Congress Cataloging in Publication Data
Timms, Lisa A.
    60 social situations and discussion starters to help teens on the autism spectrum deal
with friendships, feelings, conflict and more : seeing the big picture / Lisa A. Timms.
        p. cm.
    ISBN 978-1-84905-862-9 (alk. paper)
    1. Autism in adolescence. 2. Social skills in adolescence. 3. Autistic youth--Life
skills guides. I. Title. II. Title: Sixty social situations and discussion starters to help
teens on the autism spectrum deal with friendships, feelings, conflict and more.
    RJ506.A9T55 2011
    618.92'85882--dc22
                                    2010052929

British Library Cataloguing in Publication Data
A CIP catalogue record for this book is available from the British Library

ISBN 978 1 84905 862 9

Printed and bound in Great Britain

Contents

Acknowledgments

There are many people I would like to thank who have helped me with the creation of this book. I would like to thank my son Cody Timms for being so supportive and patient while I was working on the publication process. He is seriously the best kid ever! I would like to thank my friend Joann Pesavento-Dudick for never losing faith in me and always telling me to believe in my dreams. The law of attraction works! I would like to thank Carla Romanchick for her comic relief. I would like to thank Teri Aviles, Heather Canfield, and Mary MacAderra for being so positive and supportive. I would like to thank my friend Karla Beadle for being one of the most optimistic people I have ever met. I would like to thank Cindy Loftus-Vergari and Donna Podrazik for their positive reinforcement. I would like to thank Dr. Charles Glean for giving me the opportunity to start the social skills program, his guidance and having faith in me throughout the process. I would like to thank Judy Deemer, Heidi Gardner, and Maryann Johnson, for being my friends and for truly listening to my ideas and giving caring and compassionate feedback in both my professional and personal life. I would like to thank Alison Potter, and Jen Alberti for not only being caring co-workers but also for being my friends and giving both me and the social skills program the support I so needed at times. I would like to thank Lisa Slover for probably being my biggest fan. I would like to thank Joe Monichelli for his help with the original book proposal. The timing was impeccable. I would like to thank everyone I have worked with at Jessica Kingsley Publishers for giving me the opportunity to share my situations with other teens and their parents that I would not be able to reach otherwise. Finally I would like to thank all my students and their parents who made the social skills program and this book possible in the first place. Every student I have ever worked with is absolutely awesome! Every person mentioned in this dedication has gone above and beyond for me. I thank you all with all my heart!

Introduction

Individuals with Autism Spectrum Disorder (ASD) see the world very differently than the average person. Individuals with ASD think very literally. They have a hard time understanding sarcasm and idioms. If someone with ASD asks you if you would like to go see a movie you really want to see and you sarcastically answer "I do not want to see *that* movie" the individual with ASD will think you really do not want to see that movie and suggest a different movie. When you tell them you were kidding they may look at you like you are lying to them. If you tell someone with ASD "Let's go out and paint the town red!" that individual may think they need to go to the store and buy red paint and paint brushes to prepare for your evening out. Almost everything is black or white; they have a difficult time seeing the "grey area" in anything. Individuals with ASD also have a hard time "putting themselves in someone else's shoes." They find it very difficult to see something from someone else's point of view. The situations included in this book help these individuals (especially teens) work through different situations they may encounter. It gives them the opportunity to try to see someone else's point of view. It gives them a safe time to honestly discuss how they would approach different situations. This gives the person working with them the opportunity to explain why others may find their response inappropriate and help them reach a socially acceptable response.

How to use this book

This book was designed with both the teen and the parent in mind. The sections are not in any specific order. Feel free to skip around and pick the topic your teen might be having issues with. I suggest you read the situation with your teen and do the discussion questions together. You could write your responses down and compare them with your teen's responses. Even if your teen gives you a seemingly incorrect response please do not tell them they are wrong. Ask them why they responded to the question the way they did. The majority of the time your teen will have a legitimate reason for their response. It will give you insight into how your teen processes information and how they think about different situations. You may be surprised!

The parent homework is designed to help you generalize the skill into the "real world." The best way to gain insight into your teen is through communication. Each parent homework assignment involves communicating with your teen in some way and relating the skill to a time when the teen has experienced the topic in real life. Nothing generalizes a skill more than putting it into perspective with something your teen has gone through. Try to keep it light and related to the topic. I hope these situations help your teen as much as they have helped my students. Enjoy!

Chapter 1

Self-Esteem

Why are we talking about this?

Individuals with ASD sometimes struggle with self-esteem issues. This is due to them not completely understanding why others do not act or say things the same way they do. They know they are different and sometimes this is hard for them to accept. This chapter helps them work through various self-esteem issues.

What is Encouragement? This is Too Hard!

Joey has been watching the science fiction series *Comet Battle* for as long as he can remember. He is a huge fan. He owns every movie and can recite most of the dialogue by heart. His parents decided to get him the Ultimate Collectors Cosmos kit for his birthday. When Joey opened it he was so excited! It was the biggest collector's kit ever made with over 5000 pieces! He could not wait to get started! He immediately opened the box and looked at the directions. There were a lot of directions, over 100 pages. Joey carefully sorted out the pieces and started at Step 1.

Joey did well until Step 25. He was supposed to connect two larger pieces but he just could not figure out how to do it. He looked at the picture over and over. Was he missing something? Joey became very discouraged. He threw the directions down and went to his room. His older brother Sid came up to see what was wrong. Sid was in college and Joey thought he was very intelligent. Joey explained how he felt stupid because he could not get past Step 25. Sid asked him if he would like some help. Joey said "yes."

Joey and Sid went back downstairs and looked over the directions again. As far as Sid could tell, Joey had done everything right so far and he could not figure out why the parts were not going together. They both worked on the project for about 20 minutes. Finally, Sid looked at Joey and said "You know, this is not an easy thing to put together. You did a great job so far! I do not know if I would have finished this much as fast as you did. You are really good at building! We should wait until Dad has time and ask him if he could help us out."

Discussion questions

- Do you think Joey actually read the directions carefully or do you think he just glanced at them and tried to put the kit together?

- When Joey started having problems at Step 25, do you think he went back over the directions to make sure he did not make a mistake?

- Why did Joey go to his room when he got upset?

- How do you think Joey felt when Sid offered to help him?

- How do you think Joey felt when Sid could not put it together either?

- Do you think what Sid said to Joey made him feel better?

- Do you think Joey ever went back and tried to put the kit together again?

Are these people being encouraging?

- "I noticed you received a D on your paper. You really messed that one up!"

- "It is OK if you did not make the cheerleading squad this year. There is always next year."

- "You are going to try that trick again? Why would you want to do that? You are only going to fall again and this time you might really hurt yourself!"

- I know you have been trying to land that trick. Keep practicing. You will get it."

- "You have been working so hard on your project. I know it has been difficult. You are already half way done! Way to go!"

Parent homework

I "encourage" you to talk to your teen about a time when you were completely discouraged and someone consoled you and made you feel better. Your teen will realize that even parents felt better from a kind word at one time. You will be amazed at the impact that can have. When you encourage your teen, use the word "encourage" to help them clearly understand the word and the actions behind it.

The Importance of Having a Sense of Humor: The Haircut

Jett was staying at Mike's house for the evening. His other friend Steve stopped by. Steve had just purchased a new set of clippers and he was dying to try them out on someone. Jett needed a haircut and decided to let Steve trim his hair. Steve decided to get a little creative and clipped some designs into Jett's hair. Steve trimmed a star, a swirl, and some diamonds into Jett's hair. Before Steve had a chance to actually trim Jett's hair to a normal style his mom called and told him he had to go home. Steve packed up his clippers and went home. Jett was left with all the different designs cut into his hair. It was late in the evening and there was nowhere he could get his hair fixed so he was stuck with the designs until the next day.

Mike got invited to a party and asked Jett to go with him. Jett really wanted to go to the party. A lot of his friends would be there. He decided to put on a hat and go to the party.

When he got to the party Mike decided to tell Jett's friends why he was wearing a hat. Ella walked up to Jett, took the hat off his head, and started to laugh so loudly that she got the attention of most of the people at the party. Now everyone was looking at Jett's head! He tried to explain what had happened but everyone at the party started laughing at him and he could not get a word in to explain. Jett got mad, left the party, and went home.

When he walked into his house his mother saw his hair and started yelling at him. She asked him why he would do something like that to his hair. Then she told him that he had to get it fixed the next day because he looked ridiculous. Jett went to his room and slammed the door.

Discussion questions

- Should Jett have let Steve experiment on his hair?

- Do you think Steve intentionally gave Jett a bad haircut?

- What could Jett have done when everyone at the party started laughing at him?

- Do you think if Jett made jokes about his haircut he still would have felt the need to leave the party?

- Do you think if Jett would have explained to his mother what happened that she still would have been angry?

Are these people showing their sense of humor?

- Lisa dropped her ice cream all over the sidewalk. Cody started laughing. Lisa smiled and went back and got another ice cream.

- Lisa dropped her ice cream all over the sidewalk. Cody started laughing. Lisa turned and yelled at Cody "It is not funny!"

- Judy was walking with Alison and fell into mud. Judy sat up and the front of her shirt and pants were completely covered in mud. Alison started to giggle while she was helping Judy up. Judy started laughing and pulled Alison into the mud.

- Judy was walking with Alison and fell into mud. Judy sat up and the front of her shirt and pants were completely covered in mud. Alison started to giggle while she was helping Judy up. Judy stood up and harshly told Alison she wished Alison had fallen into the mud instead of her.

Parent homework

Having a sense of humor about stressful things in everyday life can make the difference between having a good day and a horrible day. Talk to your teen about a time when something embarrassing happened to you and you managed to laugh it off. Some examples could be wearing a horrible bridesmaid dress or wearing two different colored socks to work. Explain how it changed the dynamic of your day. Your mindset can truly make the difference to whether you decide to enjoy the day or sit in your room and remain upset. Try to maintain a good sense of humor with your teen so you can model the skill. Also try to find humor in everyday occurrences.

Common Sense: My Computer Died!

Jesse had a desktop computer that he used all the time. He was online playing games, charging his music player, doing research for school, chatting with friends, looking at cars, or just surfing the web. If he was not out with his friends he was on the computer.

One day Jesse needed to go online to look for parts for his bike. His crank had snapped yesterday while he was riding and he wanted to see if he could find a new one online cheaper than the store price. He tried to log on to his computer but nothing was coming up on the screen. Jessie wiggled the mouse and hit the power button a few times and still nothing happened.

Jesse decided to call the computer manufacturer to see if they could help. He really needed to research the price for the crank so he could get his bike fixed. When he was connected to technical support the technician started to ask Jesse a question but before he had a chance to get the question out Jesse started complaining that he had tried everything and nothing was working. He said how lousy the computer was and just started yelling at the technician. Once Jesse stopped complaining the technician started asking him questions. The first question the technician asked Jesse was if the computer was plugged in. Jesse replied "What, do you think I am stupid or something?! Of course I checked to see if the computer was plugged in!" Next the technician asked Jesse if the computer was plugged into an outlet or a power strip. Jesse told him it was plugged into a power strip. Then the technician asked Jesse if the power strip was turned on. Jesse looked and the power strip was turned off. He had no idea how it got turned off but it was off nonetheless. Jesse apologized to the technician, turned on the power strip and the computer worked fine.

He was telling his friend David what had happened. David started laughing and said "Way to use common sense, Jesse!"

Discussion questions

- What do you think common sense is?

- How do you think others view you if you lack common sense?

- How do you think common sense relates to self-esteem?

- In what other way could Jesse have found prices for the crank other than using the computer?

- What should Jesse have done when he called the technician instead of complaining about the computer?

- How do you think Jesse felt when he realized the power strip was turned off?

- What do you think David meant when he said "Way to use common sense"?

Are these people using common sense?

- It was cold outside and started to rain. Jeremy stayed out in the rain and complained that he was cold instead of coming into the house.

- Pat saw a television on sale. The advertisement said the television was on sale for $250. Pat went to the store to purchase the television with $225.

- Steve was learning tricks on his bike. His coach told him not to practice on loose dirt or gravel since it would kick out the tires. Steve saw a patch of gravel and did not try the trick in the gravel.

- Mike's computer lost internet connection. Mike checked and saw the cord was unplugged from the back of the computer. Mike plugged the cord back in.

- Karla was supposed to sign up for training at work. She did not clearly understand the directions. She signed up for the wrong training.

Parent homework

We have all had a momentary lapse in common sense at one point in time in our lives. Whether it was trying to figure out why the car would not start and then realizing you are out of gas or spending the day in the sun when you forgot your sunscreen and got sunburn. It happens to everyone. Talk to your teen about a time when you had a lapse in common sense and made a simple mistake that common sense would have solved. Your teen will know it happens to everyone and it is no reason to feel bad. Use everyday situations to practice common sense skills. Even though something may seem obvious to you it may not be as obvious to your teen.

Your Opinion Matters: The Road Trip

Joann, Heather, Scott, and Jamie were planning a road trip. They all wanted to go on a trip for the upcoming weekend but they could not decide where to go. While Joann, Heather, and Scott were talking about different places to go Jamie sat quietly. When they asked Jamie if he had any ideas he said he did not care where they went. Jamie thought his opinion did not matter. The others decided to go to a water park.

The next decision was a little more difficult. Which park to go to? There were four major parks within a two-hour drive. After some discussion they decided to go to Hot Point Water Park. None of them had ever been there before and the online brochure looked good. They left on Saturday morning and headed for the park.

When they got there the place was a mess! Most of the rides were shut down due to maintenance issues. The ones that were open had very long lines. The wave pool had stuff floating in it and kept breaking down. Everyone was miserable! Why did they decide to go to Hot Point?

On the way home they stopped for dinner. During dinner Jamie said they should have gone to Cool Tides Water Park. Heather said they could not go there because the park was not even open yet. The grand opening was in two weeks. Jamie said he was a member of waterparks. com and he had received an email a week ago about the park. Because he was a member of the site he could get into the park two weeks before the public grand opening. He also could get up to four friends in for a discounted price during the promotion.

Scott, Joann, and Heather all looked at Jamie. Scott asked Jamie why he did not say anything when they were trying to decide where to go. Jamie said he did not say anything because he did not care where they went. Then Joann told Jamie that they had not known they could get into the park before the grand opening and that if they had known they definitely would have gone there.

Everyone was upset with Jamie but he did not know why. He told them he did not care where they went. He was wondering how it was his fault that they had such a horrible Saturday.

Discussion questions

- Why did Jamie not mention anything when everyone was deciding where to go for the weekend?

- Why do you think Jamie thought his opinion did not matter?

- Why do you think everyone got mad at Jamie after he told them about Cool Tides Water Park?

- Do you think if Jamie had told them about Cool Tides Water Park that they would have gone there?

- Do you think they still would have been mad at Jamie if they decided not to go to Cool Tides Water Park after he told them about it?

Would their opinion matter to you?

- You are looking forward to having your birthday party in your back yard. You have all sorts of games and activities planned that can only be done outside. Your friend asks why you are having the party in the back yard since it would be more fun to have it at the lodge.

- You are unsure what movie to see this weekend. There are two movies playing in the theatre that you are interested in. Your friend tells you to see one of the movies. They have already seen the movie and said it was excellent.

- You are going to buy a new cell phone. You have done research for weeks and finally decided on which phone to get. You really like the phone you have decided to purchase. Your friend tells you the phone you picked is too cheap and tells you to purchase a more expensive phone.

- You are going on vacation and you are trying to choose a hotel. You just started looking at different places to stay. Your friend tells you about a hotel on the beach they stayed at last year with great views and three pools.

- You have decided to go snow tubing with a group of friends. There are three different slopes within an hour's drive. One of your friends suggests a slope that is four hours away.

Parent homework

There are times when your teen might be afraid to speak up when asked their opinion on something. Whether they are asked about somewhere to go or if a friend asks them if they look OK in a horrible outfit kids can feel uncomfortable stating their opinion. Talk to your teen about how to tactfully give an opinion. If someone asks them where they would like to go they can tell them. The worst that could happen is the group decides to go somewhere else. Explain to your teen that that would not be a reflection on them personally; it would just be that the others made a different decision. If it is about a bad wardrobe choice ask your teen how they would feel if they asked someone how they looked when they looked horrible and then went out in public like that. Giving a suggestion or an honest opinion is not a bad thing as long as it is given thoughtfully.

Strengths: Everyone is Good at Something

Raina and her friends all hung out at the local community center. Three days out of the week the community center would have different activities for the kids. Monday was dance, Wednesday was swimming, and on Friday they did different craft projects. Raina refused to participate in the different activities and her friends were always trying to talk her into going. They kept telling her "Try it you might like it!" but Raina just kept saying no.

One weekend Raina invited her friend Zack to come to her house and offered to make him lunch. She decided to try a new recipe she had been working on. While they were eating lunch Zack asked her why she would not go to any of the activities. He told her how much fun he was having. He told her about Monday's dance activity and how he did not feel comfortable doing it but he had a great time watching everyone else. Then he told her about Wednesday's swim activity where all the kids went diving for tokens. The people with the top three amounts of tokens won prizes. Then he told her about Friday's craft activity. They all got to build feeders for chipmunks.

Raina told Zack she was not good at anything. She could not dance at all because she could not keep a beat. She did not know how to swim and she thought the other kids would make fun of her. She did not want to go to the craft class because she was afraid she would not be able to do what they wanted her to do. Raina was really depressed. She wanted to spend time with her friends but she did not want all of them to know she was not good at anything.

Zack looked at Raina and started laughing. Raina got very upset and yelled at Zack not to laugh at her. Zack apologized and said he could not believe she thought she was not good at anything! Zack told her every time she had invited him over for lunch or dinner the food was fantastic. She was probably the best cook he knew! How in the world could she think she was not good at anything? She was always coming up with new recipes and trying them out on Zack. She had yet to make anything he did not like. He told her that she should talk to the community center and see if they would start a cooking class.

Discussion questions

- Why do you think Raina thought she was not good at anything?

- Why do you think Zack laughed at Raina when she told him she was not good at anything?

- Do you think Raina's friends would think differently of her if they knew she was not good at the community center activities?

- Do you think all of Raina's friends were good at all of the activities?

- What would you have done if you were Raina?

- How would you try to talk her into trying new things?

- Do you think Raina would have fun if she went to the activities?

Examples of talents

Various sports	Mechanics
Academics	Cooking
Being business minded	Singing
Fashion sense	Being a good friend
Musical instruments	Helping others
Problem solving	Sewing

Can you think of other talents?

Parent homework

Everyone is good at something. Absolutely everyone has a talent. Sometimes it is just not obvious to that person what their talent is and you have to point it out to them. Ask your teen to make a list of what they think their talents are and you also make a list of what you think your teen's talents are. Then sit down and compare lists. You might be surprised to see that your teen does not recognize all of their strengths. Explain to your teen that strength could be obvious like being great at a sport or subtle like being a good conversationalist. Help your teen nurture their talents. Who knows, someday their talent might turn into a career!

Chapter **2**

Problem Solving

Why are we talking about this?

General problem solving can be an issue for individuals with ASD. They see things literally so when they are faced with a problem they sometimes think everything has a yes or no answer. This chapter helps them think of different solutions to various problems.

What Could I Do? Getting to Practice

Jeff had a basketball game at his school. It was a very important game because his team were in second place and was playing the first place team. If they won, they would go to the divisional playoffs! Jeff was the point guard for the team; he was one of the best players they had and it would be difficult to win the game without him.

Jeff had been preparing for this game for weeks. He practiced every day with his friends at the local basketball court. He knew he was ready. He would not let his team down.

Jeff and his mother got into the car to leave for the game. The car would not start! Jeff's mother kept trying but with no luck. The car just would not start.

Jeff got very angry. He started yelling about the car being a lousy car, he got out and slammed the door and kicked the side of the car. What was he going to do now? The game started in an hour. Not going was not an option. He started yelling at his mother asking her how could this happen today of all days!

He saw how upset this made his mother. He apologized to his mother and asked her what he should do. If his team lost because he was not there they would never forgive him. Everyone in school would be mad at him. This was their chance at being number one in the division.

Jeff's mother told him to take a deep breath. She said they would figure something out. Then Jeff's mother looked at him and asked him if he could think of any solutions.

Discussion questions

- Do you think Jeff's mother wanted the car to break down?

- Do you think Jeff had the right to be upset?

- Do you think Jeff's team mates would understand if he did not make it to the game?

- Do you think Jeff had other options other than not going to the game?

- What would you do if you were Jeff?

How would you solve this problem?

- You promised your friend you would go shopping with them today but you hurt your ankle and could not walk.

- Your dog actually ate your homework.

- You want to go swimming at a friend's house but you do not have a ride there.

- It is very hot outside and your air conditioner just broke.

- You woke up and found out the water main broke in front of your house and you have no water.

Parent homework

Talk to your teen and create different problem scenarios such as being out of milk for breakfast to missing a big test at school and various other scenarios in between. Ask your teen to rate them from most important to least important (this will give you a good gauge on what your teen feels is important). Then discuss different solutions to the various problems.

Asking for Help Politely: I Need Help!

Brenda's teacher gave the class an assignment. Brenda was having a hard time with the assignment. The teacher verbally gave the directions. Brenda did not completely understand the directions. She thought about what the teacher said over and over. Did she miss something? She became very frustrated. She wanted to ask for help but she did not know who to ask. She asked one student for the answers and they told her to figure it out herself. Then she asked another student and they completely ignored her. Finally, she decided to ask the teacher.

By the time Brenda decided to ask the teacher she was very upset. She walked up to the teacher and yelled "I do not understand this. It is stupid! Why do we have to do this in the first place?"

The teacher gave Brenda a look. The teacher understood that Brenda needed help but she was not happy about the way Brenda asked. The teacher asked "What seems to be the problem?"

Brenda again said the assignment was stupid and she did not want to do it. The teacher calmly asked Brenda to sit down and think about what she really wanted. When she was ready she could come back to the teacher and ask.

Brenda went back to her desk and just sat there. Did not the teacher understand that she did not know what to do? Why would the teacher not just help her?

Discussion questions

- Do you think Brenda could have done the assignment on her own?

- Do you think if Brenda wrote down the directions it would have been easier for her to understand the assignment?

- Do you think if Brenda asked the first student for help with the directions instead of asking for the answers she would have received a different response?

- What would have been a better way for Brenda to ask the teacher for help?

Are these people asking for help politely?

- "I could not put this puzzle together. Would you please help me?"

- "This part will not come off my bike! Get over here and help me!"

- "My video game does not seem to be working. Can you help me figure out why?"

- "I cannot remember what page we were supposed to do for homework. Do you remember the page number?"

- "I forgot to do my homework again. Give me your paper right now so I can copy the answers."

Parent homework

Sometimes we need help from our teen. The next time you request your teen's assistance with something, do it in a polite manner. After they respond positively, show them an inappropriate way to ask for help. Ask them if they would have been as willing to lend a hand if you had asked impolitely first. Modeling the skill will help your teen understand what an appropriate way to ask is.

Who Can Help You: How Do You Do That?

Chelsea was the best skateboarder in town. She was even better than the boys! The tricks came easily to her. It seemed that all she had to do was see a trick done once and she could pick it up. Everyone came to her for help when they wanted to learn something new. One day Chelsea was watching a new skateboarding video she had just bought. One of the skateboarders landed a 1080 (three complete spins in the air before landing). Chelsea tried and tried but just could not get this trick down. She stopped skating with her friends.

Chelsea's best friend Sean called and asked Chelsea where she had been. No one had seen her and they missed skating with her. Chelsea told Sean why she had not been skating. Sean told Chelsea that his cousin Tony was coming in this weekend to visit. He really wanted Chelsea to meet him. Chelsea still felt embarrassed but she went to meet Tony. Chelsea skated with Tony and Sean for a while. Tony told her how impressed he was with all the tricks she could do. Sean told Tony about Chelsea having problems with the 1080 she was trying to land.

Chelsea was upset that Sean even brought that up. She did not want everyone to know she just could not do it. What Chelsea did not realize was that Tony was the skater in the video doing the 1080! Tony told her he could help. He walked her through the steps and explained how to do it. After three tries she got it! Tony was actually able to help Chelsea learn the trick! She had been asked to help other people learn things all the time but she never had to ask for help. She was so happy Sean talked her into meeting Tony!

Discussion questions

- Why do you think Chelsea would not hang out with her friends when she could not do the trick?

- Do you think Chelsea's friends would have thought any less of her if they knew she could not do the trick?

- Why do you think Sean wanted Chelsea to meet Tony?

- Do you think Tony thought Chelsea was a lousy skateboarder because she could not do the trick?

- How do you think Sean felt when Tony was able to teach Chelsea the trick?

- How do you think Chelsea felt when she realized she could ask for help?

How can these people help you?

- A family member.
- Your best friend.

- A neighbor.

- A favorite teacher.

- A counselor.

- A police officer.

- A fireman.

Parent homework

Talk to your teen about situations they might get into where they would have to ask for help. This is the perfect opportunity to cover some sensitive topics. I would suggest covering the following:

- homework and/or schoolwork

- learning something new

- problems they may not be able to talk to you about

- if they are lost or a stranger approaches them

- how different people can help with different situations.

Waiting Out a Problem: This Too Shall Pass

Danielle was an amazing artist. She was looking forward to the arts festival which was happening the upcoming weekend. The festival was to be held on Friday, Saturday, and Sunday. She had five pieces that were going to be displayed during the festival. She was so excited. Maybe she would even sell one of her pieces! She could not wait!

On Thursday evening Danielle sat down to see what the weather was going to be like for the weekend. The weatherman said a tropical storm was coming up the coast and it would rain from Friday to Monday. Danielle was so upset! She had been looking forward to the festival for months, ever since she was invited to display her pieces. Her mood turned from happy to miserable in a matter of seconds.

Danielle's brother Billy came home from work and asked Danielle if she was ready for the festival at the weekend. He did not know what the weather was going to be like that weekend. Danielle yelled back at Billy telling him he was a jerk and saying how could he ask her that? She went up to her room and slammed the door. Billy looked at his mom and asked "What is up with her?!"

Billy's mom explained that Danielle was upset because of the weather. The festival would have to be postponed for another month. Billy did not know but he felt horrible about bringing it up to Danielle. He did not want to hurt her feelings, and he knew how much she was looking forward to the festival.

Billy went up to Danielle's room to talk to her. She was lying on her bed watching TV. He told her he was sorry for asking but he did not know it was going to be postponed. He tried to comfort her by telling her it was just another month that she would have to wait. He told her the pieces she did were fantastic and anyone would be happy to purchase them. Danielle calmed down a little. Billy looked at her and said "This too shall pass."

Discussion questions

- Do you think Danielle had a right to be upset about the festival being postponed?

- What would you have done if you were Danielle?

- How do you think Billy felt when Danielle yelled at him when he asked her if she was ready for the festival?

- What do you think Billy meant when he said "This too shall pass"?

Do you think these problems can be solved just by waiting?

- You need to get something at the store but your parents are busy right now. They said they will take you to the store when they are done.

- You have an appointment at 1pm. You wanted to be there early but you missed the bus. The next bus will get you to your appointment right at 1pm.

- You slept in for school. You have a test first period. Your brother said he will take you to school after he does some work around the house. Your sister said she will take to you to school immediately.

- You got into an argument with your best friend. You are still friends but things just do not seem the same.

- Your friend moved away. You do not know when you will be able to see them again. You are really upset.

Parent homework

There are situations that happen that we have no control over. Things such as the weather are an obvious one. No matter how hard we try we cannot change the weather. There are problems your teen may encounter that just need to be waited out. Sometimes time is the best solution for something. If your teen failed a test you can console them by saying they will do better on the next one and the feelings they are currently feeling will fade over time. The saying works well when your teen is feeling something that you know will lessen over time. If your teen understands that time heals most wounds it can help them calm down a bit and work through the intense feelings they may be experiencing. Talk them through it and remind them…this too shall pass.

Decision Making: Homebound or Schoolbound

Nate was a senior who hated school. He did not like any of his teachers and did not have any of his friends in his classes. On top of this Nate suffered from stress-induced migraines so at times if he got upset he would get sick.

Nate decided he would change to the homebound program. Homebound is when the teacher comes to your house and goes over your lessons with you. He did not think his parents would approve of it so he decided to come up with a plan. He researched the program and presented it to his parents with a lot of enthusiasm and information. Much to his surprise they agreed. They felt that he put a lot of time and effort into finding out all the information and it would probably be best for him.

Nate's parents took him to the doctor and had all of the necessary paperwork filled out for homebound instruction. Nate was so relieved. He would not have to put up with the teachers he did not like anymore. He would be able to get his work done at home and still graduate with his friends. He was excited to begin the program.

The school called Nate's parents to tell them who his teacher would be. Nate was assigned Ms. Smith. When Nate's parents told him who he had he became very upset. He really hated Ms. Smith. She had been one of his teachers in the past and she was really tough on him. She was a former drill sergeant who did not put up with anything. Nate had argued with her before and had got into trouble. She did not understand him at all. What was he going to do now?

Nate told his parents he wanted to go back to school. His parents explained that it was too late. He already had a note from the doctor stating that he was unable to attend school so homebound was the only option. Nate threatened to quit school if he had to have Ms. Smith as his teacher. His parents told him that was not an option and he would have to find a way to make it work. Nate could not decide what other options he might have.

Discussion questions

- Do you think it was a good idea for Nate to suggest homebound instruction to his parents?

- Do you think Nate could have found a way to make going to school work for him?

- Do you think Nate had other choices besides homebound instruction?

- Do you think Nate is going to get along with Ms. Smith when they meet for instruction?

- Does Nate have any other options?

- What would you do if you were Nate? Can you come up with other solutions?

Look at the following examples and try to make the best decision

- You have $20 for the weekend. You could go to a movie or go out to eat with friends but you do not have enough money for both. What would you do?

- You have a part-time job that you love but you do not make enough money. You are offered another part-time job for more money but you do not think you will enjoy it as much. The hours conflict and you could not work both jobs. What would you do?

- Your car broke down on a back road and you have no cell phone reception. There are no pay phones around. What would you do?

- You are due for an upgrade on your cell phone but the phone you want will cause your monthly bill to increase. Your parents told you they will not pay any extra for your cell phone bill. What would you do?

- There are two electives that you want to take in school this year. They are offered on the same day at the same time. How would you decide which one to choose?

Parent homework

Sometimes teens are forced to make some difficult decisions. Even if they do all the research and think they are making the best choice it could backfire on them. If your teen is faced with a decision, help them gather as much information as you can so they can make an informed decision. Sometimes they need to make a decision quickly. Help your teen think through what would be the best thing to do. We cannot predict what types of situations our teens will get into day by day. We can only help them by teaching them how to analyze a problem, think up possible different solutions, and then choose the one that works best for them. Try to be supportive in the decisions your teen makes on their own. If the decision does not go the way they expected, talk to them and guide them to finding possible solutions for the difficult problems. As parents, we need to do the best we can to support our teens and help them make good decisions.

Chapter **3**

Friendships

Why are we talking about this?

Individuals with ASD sometimes have a hard time making and maintaining friendships. This could be due to various issues such as: not understanding personal space, not understanding someone else's point of view, not understanding what type of question is too personal to ask, etc. This chapter goes through various situations a teen may encounter involving friends and gives them the opportunity to work through them.

Asking Personal Questions: Hard Times

Arley and Emma were close friends. They knew just about everything about each other. Arley lived with her aunt and uncle while Emma lived with her parents. Both the girls' families were very close to each other. Emma's mom talked to Arley's aunt almost every day. One day Arley was very upset. Emma asked her what was wrong. Arley went on to explain that her uncle had lost his job due to the company closing and they were having financial problems. Emma went home and told her mom but she already knew. Arley's aunt had called her that morning and told her what happened.

Emma's family really wanted to help Arley's family get through this difficult time. Emma's mom said she would give Arley's family some clothing that no longer fitted her children. Emma's mom also went to the store and bought groceries for Arley's family to help out a little.

Arley and Emma always stuck together. One day, Arley was at the mall with Emma wearing one of Emma's outfits that her mom had given her. Sadie, a girl from down the street, walked up to them. Sadie did not have many friends and she wanted to hang out with Arley and Emma. Sadie walked up to Arley and said "Why are you wearing Emma's old clothes? Does not your family buy you clothes?"

Arley got very upset and started to cry. Emma started yelling at Sadie and calling her "nosey," "stuck up," and "mean." Emma ran after Arley to make sure she was OK.

Sadie could not understand why everyone was so upset with her. Why was it every time she asked someone a question they got mad at her?

Discussion questions

- How do you think Arley felt when her uncle lost his job?

- Was it OK for Emma to ask Arley what was wrong?

- How do you think Arley felt when she heard Emma's mom was giving her Emma's old clothes?

- How do you think Emma felt about it?

- Was it OK for Sadie to ask Arley why she was wearing Emma's old clothes?

- Do you think Emma was right for calling Sadie names?

- Why do you think Sadie does not have many friends?

- What would you have done if you were:
  - Arley?
  - Emma?
  - Sadie?

Do you think this is a personal question?

- How old are you?

- How much do you weigh?

- How much money do your parents make?
- What is your name?
- What do you like to do?

Parent homework

When we were children we have all asked someone a personal question. Whether it was something as simple as asking an older woman her age or asking someone how much they weigh. As kids, it is hard to understand why people would be upset by these questions. They certainly seem innocent enough. Think about topics you are sensitive about and talk to your teen about them. Explain to them that certain questions do not bother you but others do. Also explain that everyone is different and just because you might be OK with telling your age that does not mean that everyone else is. Explain to your teen that not crossing the line with people you do not know is always difficult. If they are unsure about a question do not ask. If they ask and seemingly offend someone, immediately apologize, change the subject, and do not ask that person that question again.

Friends with Friends: Why Are You Helping Her?

Halee and Mackenzie were very close friends. They spent a lot of time together. They saw each other every day at school and then they hung out together after school. They were practically inseparable. They had another friend Ciara who would sometimes come over to watch movies or just hang out.

Ciara's birthday was coming up soon. She knew exactly how she wanted her party to go. She asked her mom if she could plan the party. Her mom said OK.

Ciara was closer to Mackenzie than to Halee. She asked Mackenzie to help her plan the party. They needed to make a guest list and purchase the invitations, decorations, party favors, and snacks. There was so much to plan!

Halee felt really left out. Instead of Mackenzie spending every day with her she seemed too busy with Ciara's party to do anything. Every time Halee called Mackenzie she was going somewhere with Ciara. Halee started to strongly dislike Ciara.

Then Halee started acting weird toward Mackenzie. She stopped taking her calls and avoided her when she saw her out. Halee was invited to the party but she told Mackenzie she was not going to go. Mackenzie was upset. She had spent so much time planning the party and she really wanted her best friend there.

Discussion questions

- What would you have done if you were Halee?
- Would you have treated Mackenzie differently?
- Would you have gone to Ciara's birthday party?
- What would you have done if you were Mackenzie?
- How could you make Halee feel better?

What would you do?

- Your friend is upset because he or she thinks you are not spending enough time with them.
- Your best friend decides to go to a movie you wanted to see with someone else and does not invite you.
- Your friend is upset because they want you to help them but you are too busy helping another friend.
- You have a problem and you call your friend but they tell you they are with someone else and will call you back later.
- You send a text to your friend asking them to meet you at the park and they do not respond. You then see them at the park with a different friend.

Parent homework

If your teen is the one upset because they feel like they are getting slighted talk to them about their feelings. They are valid feelings to your teen. Explain how they might some day have to make a difficult decision between friends and ask them how they would like their friends to treat them regarding the decision they make.

Conflicting Events: You Are Going Where?

Bastian was a very popular kid. He had all sorts of friends. He hung out with the bikers, the skateboarders, the jocks, and the intellectual kids. He was friends with everyone!

Because he had such a wide variety of friends he always had conflicting events. There was so much to do! He wanted to keep it fair so he tried to take turns between the groups.

One day there was a skateboarding event happening at the same time as a biking event. Bastian always helped his friends at the events. He was great at fixing things so he would go and set up their gear and fix anything that might break during the event.

He decided to go to the biking event. His favorite pro biker was going to be there. He was so excited! He might actually meet him!

When he told the skaters he was not going to their event a few of them started calling him names and being very mean. They said he was a jerk for blowing them off. Bastian could not understand why they were so angry.

Discussion questions

- What would you have done if you were Bastian?
- Would you still have gone to the biking event?
- What would you have said to the skaters?
- What would you do if you were one of the skaters?
- Would you stay angry at Bastian for not going to the event?

What would you do?

- Your best friend invites you to go to a movie but your boyfriend/girlfriend invites you to go to dinner.
- You have already made plans to go to a party with your friend but another friend asks you to go to an amusement park that you really want to go to.
- You are out with your friend and your team mates invite you to play a game. Your friend does not play the sport.

- Three different friends ask you to do something on Saturday night.

- You are at the mall with your friend and another friend wants you to help them find an outfit to wear for the weekend.

Parent homework

It can be difficult for kids to understand that they are not the only friend someone has, especially if there are conflicting plans. If this happens to your teen sit down with them and talk it out. Help them make a decision. Explain to them that they need to explain their decision to both of their friends so they understand what happened. Help them be fair if the situation arises again.

Personal Space: Getting a Bit Too Touchy

It was a cold winter day. Jaden, Missy, Abby, and Wade decided to get together to go sledding. They all grabbed their sleds and headed off to the local neighborhood park. The park had a great sledding hill. It was long and steep. Everyone was standing at the top of the hill getting ready to get on their sleds when Wade came up behind Missy and pushed her. Missy went tumbling down the hill. Wade was laughing but Missy was very upset. Next, Wade went to Jaden. Just as Jaden was getting ready to push off to go down the hill, Wade grabbed the back of his coat and Jaden stopped dead.

Abby walked up to Wade and started yelling at him. She said he was not being very nice and she thought he should go home. Wade walked up to Abby and gave her a very tight hug to apologize. This made Abby very uncomfortable and she told Wade to go home.

Wade went home very sad. He could not understand why his friends were so upset with him. He was just fooling around. He especially could not understand why Abby would get so angry over a hug. After all, it was just a hug.

Discussion questions

- Why do you think Missy was upset with Wade? (Missy is the one he pushed down the hill.)

- Why do you think Jaden was upset with Wade? (Wade grabbed Jaden's coat just as Jaden was getting ready to go down the hill.)

- Why do you think Abby yelled at Wade? He did not do anything to her.

- Why do you think the hug upset Abby?

- Do you think Abby, Jaden, and Missy will invite Wade to do anything with them again?

- Do you think Wade has a hard time keeping friends?

Are you invading personal space?

- You have just met someone and you give them a tight hug.

- You are standing in line at the store and you are six inches away from the person in front of you.

- You are talking to someone and you are three inches away from their face.

- You are standing next to someone you do not know and there is approximately 18 inches between you.

- You are near the stage at a concert and everyone is crowding together.

Parent homework

Most of us have had a friend at one time or another who was adamant about having their own space. Share a story with your teen about someone you know (or knew) who really needed their space. Tell your teen how that person would react if someone invaded their personal space. Also, explain the appropriate personal space. It is usually at least three feet all around the person.

Try this exercise. Have your teen stand with their back to the wall. Stand in front of your teen while respecting their personal space. Then, keep stepping in until you are right in their face. Ask them how they feel as you are moving closer. Even though your teen is familiar with you, it can still be uncomfortable. Then, tell your teen to imagine someone they just met doing that to them. Help them understand how invading someone's personal space can make them feel uncomfortable.

Being Trustworthy: Show Your True Colors

Celia and Jack lived next door to each other. They were the same age and in the same grade. They would frequently see each other at school, at the park, or just hanging out with their friends.

One day Celia would see Jack and be very friendly to him. They would chat and joke around. They seemed like good friends. Jack told Celia things he was embarrassed to tell his friends. He felt he could trust her.

Another day Celia would be with her other friends and see Jack. This time she would completely ignore him. She would talk to her friends and glance at him and giggle. Jack was sure Celia was telling her friends things he had told her in confidence.

This completely confused Jack. He just did not get it. Why was she acting this way? Jack wished Celia would just show her true colors already!

Discussion questions

- Do you think that Celia was nice to Jack just so she could find out things about him to tell her friends?

- Do you think Celia told her friends what Jack told her in confidence?

- Do you think Celia was really Jack's friend?

- If you were Jack would you ever tell Celia anything in confidence again?

- What would you have done if you were Jack?

- Do you think Celia was trustworthy?
- What does it mean when someone talks about your "true colors"?

Are these people showing their true colors?

- Your friend acts one way when they are with you and acts completely differently when they are around someone else.

- Someone you know says they are not prejudiced but then they say they think a certain race is inferior to their own.

- You tell everyone your friend is thoughtful and your friend helps an elderly person cross the street.

- Your friend claims to be forgiving and accepts your apology when you break their favorite collectable.

Parent homework

Talk to your teen about what trust means to them. Give them little tasks to do that require trust such as mailing a letter or doing some type of household chore. Emphasize how trustworthy they are when they complete the task (they are trustworthy because they did what they said they would do). Tell your teen what a good friend they must be because they can be trusted.

Chapter 4

Dealing with Feelings

Why are we talking about this?

Individuals with ASD sometimes have a hard time understanding their own feelings and the feelings of others. They realize others think and feel differently than they do but they are not sure how to approach it. For example, if you lost your cat and the person with ASD does not particularly like cats, they may wonder why you are upset. This chapter gives teens the opportunity to work through their feelings and how they may relate to others.

Understanding Your Feelings: The Day Care Center

Piper had a part-time job at a local day care center. This was her second year on the job and she loved it. She enjoyed spending time with the kids. She had the opportunity to play with them and also to teach them new things. Piper wanted to go to college to be a pre-school teacher so this seemed like the perfect job for her.

During Piper's first year on the job she had learned the ropes very quickly. During every training session Piper went to, she actively participated and the answers came easily to her. She was a natural working with the kids, especially the younger children. For her first year Piper was assigned to work with the pre-schoolers. She did an excellent job and her supervisor told her what a great employee she was.

During Piper's second year on the job she was reassigned to work with the older children aged six to eight. Piper did not understand why she had been taken away from the pre-schoolers. Piper decided to talk to her supervisor.

Piper's supervisor told her again what a great employee she was and how wonderful she was with the children. Her supervisor told her the decision was made to switch her to the older children because they did not feel the other staff would be able to handle the children as well as Piper did. Her supervisor told her she thought Piper would make an excellent elementary school teacher. Her supervisor told her to take it as a compliment because she did such a great job the previous year they wanted to give her a position that required more responsibility. This position was actually a promotion for Piper.

Piper went home that day and talked to her mother. She was full of emotions and needed some help sorting them out. Piper was disappointed that she would not be able to work with the pre-schoolers again this year. Her supervisor knew she wanted to be a pre-school teacher. Why would she take the experience away from her? Piper also felt honored that her supervisor thought she would be able to handle more responsibility. Piper knew she was good at her job and she was happy that her supervisor recognized it but she did not really want to work with the older children.

Piper told her best friend about the promotion at work. Her best friend told her she should be happy. It was more money and more responsibility. Piper told her best friend that her supervisor told her it was a compliment but it sure did not feel that way to Piper. Her best friend just did not understand why Piper was not happy about it.

Discussion questions

- Do you think the change in position is good for Piper?

- Why do you think Piper was not happy about receiving more responsibility at work?

- Do you think Piper had a reason for being upset over a promotion?

- How would you feel if you were Piper?

- Do you think Piper should have had a choice as to whether or not to accept the promotion instead of her supervisor just telling her what she was going to do this year?

Identify how you would feel in these situations

- Someone told your parents they saw you at a store with your friend when you were supposed to be in school.

- You just found out your father was in an accident and your brother does not seem to care at all.

- Your best friend just won an award that you wanted to win.

- You won money on a raffle ticket for the exact amount that you owe on an overdue bill.

- You got the lead role in a production and found out that you will have to perform in front of 1500 people.

Parent homework

I think we have all had mixed emotions about a situation at one time or another. We could be excited and frightened or happy and unsure all at the same time. Help your teen understand that it is OK to feel an emotion that may not be fitting for the situation. We all have the right to feel whatever emotion we are feeling at any given moment. The key is to understand why we are feeling that way and then decide how to handle our feelings. Sometimes it may mean refusing a promotion because it is not what we want. Our life experiences make us react, think, and feel the way we do. The way we perceive things are what makes us unique. If your teen is unsure about why they feel the way they do, have them make a list of the feelings they have and why they think they have them. Work through the list with your teen. It will help them understand their feelings in the future and will help them avoid feeling guilty for the way they are feeling.

Understanding How Other People Feel: Who Does Not Love Roller Coasters?

Jake loved roller coasters. As a matter of fact, he loved all rides at the amusement park. He was a thrill seeker. The faster the ride, the higher the ride, the longer the drop, the more he was excited to try it out. Jake went on a trip to an amusement park with his friend Emily. He was really excited because they had just opened up a new coaster and Jake could not wait to try it out. The problem was his friend Emily was terrified of heights and Jake did not know. When they arrived at the park the first thing Jake did was run for the new coaster. Emily followed Jake into the line.

She told Jake she was scared and she was not sure if she wanted to go on the ride. At first, Jake reassured her and told her it would be OK and she would love it. As they got closer to the ride, Emily got more and more frightened. She did not like heights, she did not like things that went fast, and she really did not like roller coasters. Jake kept trying to make Emily feel better but after a while he started to get annoyed. Jake was calling Emily a "scaredy cat" and asking her why she even came to the park in the first place if she did not want to do anything.

When it was time for them to get on the ride, Emily refused to get on the roller coaster. This made Jake pick on her even more. He yelled "How are you going to know if you like it or not if you will not even try it?"

Emily walked down the exit ramp and Jake got on the coaster. When he got off, Emily was waiting for him. He told her how great the new coaster was and how he was going to get in line to ride it again. Emily's face changed. This time she became angry. She wanted to go on rides too and the roller coaster was not one of them.

Emily started yelling at Jake and telling him if he went on the roller coaster again he was not really her friend. Jake was puzzled. Why was Emily acting like this? He loved roller coasters and everyone he knew loved roller coasters. This was one of the best roller coasters Jake had ever been on. Why could not Emily stop acting like this and just enjoy the ride like he did? Jake asked Emily, "What is the big deal?"

Discussion questions

- Do you think Jake and Emily should have felt the same way about riding the roller coaster?

- Do you think Emily should have explained to Jake why she was scared?

- Do you think it would have made a difference?

- Do you think Emily would have enjoyed the ride if she just would have tried it?

- If yes, what would you have done to convince her to ride the roller coaster?

- What would have made the whole situation better?

Is this person being understanding?

- You hate spiders and your friend finds a spider and throws it at you.

- You hate spiders and your friend grabs you and pulls you away from a huge spider.

- You say you do not know how to swim and your friend tells everyone and starts making fun of you.

- You say you do not know how to swim and your friend tells you that they will not go into the deep end of the pool.

- Your friend tells you they hate broccoli and when you have them over for dinner you tell your mom to make broccoli.

Parent homework

Think of something that you and your teen do not feel the same way about. It could be a TV show, a school subject, an activity, etc. Ask them how they feel about it, and then explain how you feel about it. Get into a discussion and justify your feelings to each other. Help your teen understand that everyone does not think/feel the same as them about everything. Keep it light.

Who is Responsible for Feelings: The Guilt Trip

Madison had an extra ticket to The Cubed Tour so she decided to invite her friend Jonathan. They had grown up together and they had the same taste in music and she thought he would really enjoy it. The Cubed Tour was a concert with 15 different bands. It was the type of music Jonathan always listened to and he could not wait to go. His all-time favorite band was going to be there too!

Madison's friend Gemma found out she had invited Jonathan to the concert. Gemma did not like that kind of music but all her other friends were going to the concert. She could not believe Madison blew her off and decided to take Jonathan instead. Gemma called Madison and told her she was not going to hang out with her anymore because she did not ask her to go to the concert. Madison tried to explain to Gemma that she did not think she would want to go since she did not listen to that type of music. She told Gemma that she asked Jonathan because she knew his favorite band would be there. She did not think Gemma would mind. Gemma did not care what Madison had to say. She was upset and felt like Madison did not think about her and continued to say things to make Madison feel bad since she did not give her extra ticket to Gemma.

Madison called Jonathan when she got off the phone with Gemma. She was so upset. She told Jonathan what Gemma had said. Jonathan told Madison that Gemma was not being very nice and that she should not let her get her so upset. Madison could not help it. Gemma was one of her best friends and she did not want her upset with her. Madison told Jonathan she did not even want to go to the concert anymore if Gemma was going to be that mad at her. Jonathan told her not to let Gemma make her feel guilty. Madison did what she thought was right and no one could make her feel guilty except for herself.

Discussion questions

- Why did Madison ask Jonathan to go to the concert instead of Gemma?

- Do you think Gemma had a right to be upset?

- How do you think Gemma could have explained her feelings better to Madison?

- Should Madison have felt guilty for asking Jonathan to the concert?

- What do you think Jonathan meant when he said that no one could make Madison feel guilty except for herself?

- Do you think Madison could have control over her feelings?

Should you feel guilty?

- You broke your mother's favorite necklace by accidentally throwing it in with the wash.

- You took your friend's car without permission and got into an accident.

- Your friend let you borrow their bike and someone stole it because you did not lock it.

- A kid in the neighborhood is picking on you and someone sticks up for you.

- You planned a trip with your friends but a snowstorm hit and now no one can go.

Parent homework

Someone once told me that guilt and worry are useless emotions. Guilt is caused by something that happened in the past that you cannot change. Worry is something that will happen in the future that you cannot change now. Either way, you have the ultimate control over how you feel. Guilt and worry are not the only emotions that your teen can learn to control. They can actually learn to control all of their emotions, both positive and negative. If you wake up in the morning and decide you are going to have a good day you will have a good day. Even if you realize what you wanted to wear has not been washed yet, if you have a positive attitude you will happily find something else to wear. It is all in your mindset. If you wake up and think it is going to be a lousy day the unlaundered outfit can put you into a rage.

Having control over your emotions is a hard concept even for adults. Practice it with your teen. When you wake up in the morning say something positive to your teen. Joke around with your teen. Make them feel like it is going to be a wonderful day and marvel at how both of you view the day differently. You truly do have more control over your emotions than you realize.

Fear and Failure: You Do Not Know Unless You Try

Lila had planned on going to Ivy University in Europe for as long as she could remember. Even when she was a little girl she would pretend she was attending the university. She would gather all her coloring books, put them into a book bag, and tell her parents she was going to her university class.

When she started grade school she told her teacher she wanted to go to Ivy University. Lila planned her courses on a college prep track (a college prep track requires the students to take courses that will help prepare them for college and/or university). She was even able to take some courses at the local community college the summer before her senior year to get a head start on her credits. Ivy University was her dream and now that she was a senior in high school, her dream could become a reality as soon as summer.

Lila had taken all of the college entrance exams and passed them with high scores. She had applied to various colleges that had her major. Even though Ivy University was her dream she decided to apply to other colleges just in case she was not accepted. She applied to local community colleges near her home, larger universities in her country, and of course she applied to Ivy University which was in a different country half-way around the world.

After a few months the acceptance letters started coming in the mail. Lila was so excited. It seemed that she had been accepted to almost every school she applied to. Lila was awaiting the letter from Ivy University. It had a reputation for only accepting the very best students and Lila wanted to become one of those students.

Lila received the letter from Ivy University. She was so nervous she could not open the letter. She asked her mother to open it for her and tell her what it said. Lila's mother opened the letter and read it to Lila. She had been accepted!

Lila's dream had come true! After the excitement of the acceptance letter wore off reality set in. Ivy University was half-way around the world. Lila had never been alone far from home. She had been on vacations but she had always had her family or friends with her. The thought of being out on her own terrified her. Would she be able to do this by herself? What would happen if she got lost in a different country? What would happen if she got there and did not like it? What would happen if she did not make any friends? What would happen if she failed a class? She talked to her parents about her fear. Lila's parents said they would be supportive of any decision Lila would make. Now all she had to do was make a decision.

Lila had thought the decision would be an easy one. After all, Ivy University was all she ever wanted. Now she was not sure what to do. She had been accepted to other colleges closer to home. Should she give in to her fear, forget about her dream and stay close to home or should she take a chance and go to Ivy University?

Discussion questions

- Do you think Lila had a good reason to be afraid to leave home?

- Do you think any of the things she was afraid of would happen to her if she left home?

- If the things she was afraid of did happen, what could she do to improve the situation?

- Do you think Lila would be completely on her own at the university?

- If you were Lila's friend, what would you say to make her feel better?

Should you face your fear?

- You are terrified of spiders and your friend wants you to hold the tarantula in science class.

- You are afraid to fly but your family is planning a trip overseas and you really want to go.

- You are in a biking competition and you want to try a new trick but you are afraid because you only got it right once.

- You do not like heights but your family wants you to go to the top of an extremely high building so you can see the city lights at night.

- You are afraid of roller coasters but your friends are trying to convince you to go on the tallest roller coaster in the world.

Parent homework

Fear can be crippling for anyone. It is difficult to watch your teen miss out on something because of fear. If you sense that your teen is avoiding something due to fear, sit down and talk with them. You can tell them about a time when you missed out on something because you were afraid to try it. It could be something as simple as a new food or something as major as a vacation. Do not accuse your teen of avoiding the activity due to fear; instead ask them why they do not want to do the activity. Your teen may or may not be honest about their fear and open up to you. No matter what your teen decides you can still help them by creating a "pro" versus "con" chart. Have them list all the positive things they would gain from the activity under "pro" and list all the negative things under "con." Help your teen decipher the list. If there are many more cons maybe it is not the correct time for your teen to face that particular fear. If there are more pros be positive about them. Remember to be supportive no matter what decision your teen makes.

Dealing with Depression: The Soccer Tryout

Hunter's father was a huge soccer fan. He even named Hunter after his favorite soccer player, Hunter Aidia. The first toy Hunter's father bought him was a soccer ball. Since the time he could walk Hunter's father was playing soccer with him.

Hunter played on soccer teams through elementary school. Hunter loved soccer almost as much as his father did but he had difficulty playing the game. He wanted to be a better player but no matter how hard he tried he just could not improve.

When Hunter got into high school he tried out for the soccer team. His high school had won the district championship the year before. Most of the players were still on the team. There were only three openings on the team and 15 players tried out. Hunter did his absolute best during the tryouts. He thought he would definitely make the team. He wanted to make his father proud.

When the list was posted showing who made the team Hunter rushed to find his name. He just knew he had made it. He had played better than he ever had before during tryouts. When he finally saw the list his name was not on it. He did not make the team. What was he going to tell his father?

Hunter went home after school and went straight to his room. After a bit, his father came into his room to ask him what was wrong. Hunter told his father he did not make the soccer team. Hunter's father looked disappointed but he told Hunter that he knew there were only a few open slots on the team. His father said it was OK that he did not make the team. It was a difficult tryout and he could always tryout again next year. Then his father turned and left his room.

Hunter became very depressed. He felt like he had let his father down. He stopped hanging out with his friends both in school and after school. His grades dropped and he was in danger of failing two of his classes. All he wanted to do was be alone in his room. He slept more than ever before. When his father asked him what was wrong Hunter yelled at him to leave him alone.

Discussion questions

- Do you think Hunter had a right to become that depressed after he did not make the soccer team?

- How would you have felt if you were Hunter and you did not make the soccer team?

- Do you think Hunter's father could have said or done something differently to make Hunter feel better about not making the team?

- What would you have said to Hunter if you were his friend and saw how upset he was?

- What could Hunter have done to make himself feel better?

What would you do?

- You feel depressed because you did not get the part in a production that you wanted. Instead of the lead role you got a supporting cast part. You have noticed you are not eating.

- You feel depressed because your dog got hit by a car and died. You had that dog since you were a little child. You really miss him. It seems all you do now is sleep.

- You feel depressed because your best friend had to move far away because their father got transferred for work. You think you are never going to see them again even though they assured you they would come back to visit when they could. You start yelling at your other friends when they ask you what is wrong.

- You feel depressed because your boyfriend/girlfriend broke up with you. Now you find yourself crying for no apparent reason and you cannot seem to make it stop. You are wondering if life is worth living without them.

- You feel depressed because you failed a class in school and now you have to go to summer school and will not be able to go on a trip that you were looking forward to. You feel like you are stupid and cannot do anything right.

Parent homework

When you are a teenager the slightest thing can put you into a depression. Teen depression can be caused by a plethora of different things. It could be puberty, a bad grade, a break-up, not making the team, someone dying, etc. For your teen it could feel like their world is crashing in around them and they do not know what to do about it.

Try to think back to when you were a teen and something happened to you that made you feel like it was the end of the world. Remember that feeling when you are trying to talk to your teen. Do not dismiss their feelings even if you think whatever they are going through is not that big a deal. To your teen it is a big deal. Have compassion for your teen. Talk to them about things that might make them feel better. Remind them of happy times they have had. If you feel that you are being ineffective with your teen suggest they talk to someone else, whether it be a friend, relative, or therapist. Sometimes no matter how hard we try we cannot make our teen feel better. That is when we need to realize that it is OK to seek outside help. Also, if you begin to feel ineffective and upset remember it is OK for you to talk to someone about your feelings too. You need to take care of yourself before you can take care of your teen.

Chapter **5**

Self-Control

Why are we talking about this?

Individuals with ASD sometimes have difficulty controlling their emotions. They can experience very intense emotions and they sometimes feel that it is OK to express them in whatever way feels appropriate at the time. This chapter gives them an opportunity to discuss various topics that may lead to a loss of self-control and work through their emotions.

Dealing with Anger and Recognizing Trigger Words: Why Would You Say That?

Tamara is a good student. She attends all of her classes, participates during class, and does all of her assignments. She gets great grades in reading and writing but she struggles with math. Tamara's friend Colin does well in math. Colin has a physical disability (he has a brace on one leg) and he cannot run or jump as well as the other kids.

Tamara was at Colin's house and they were talking about school. She told Colin that she got a D on her math paper. Colin looked at her and said "What?! Are you stupid or something? That math was easy!"

Tamara got extremely angry and lashed out at Colin. She yelled "You are a freak! You could not even walk without those stupid braces! I do not even know why I am your friend!"

Tamara left to go home and Colin was alone wondering why Tamara was so mean to him.

Discussion questions

- What did Colin say that triggered Tamara's anger?

- What was the "trigger" word?

- Why do you think she got so upset?

- What did Tamara say to Colin out of anger?

- How do you think Colin felt after Tamara said that and then left?

- What could Colin have done differently?

- What could Tamara have done differently?

- What are some things that people could say that might make you angry?

What to do if someone is angry with you

- Remain calm.

- Ask them why they are angry with you.

- Try to talk it out.

- If you are also becoming angry, walk away for a while and talk about it later.

- Some areas of sensitivity to avoid are: abilities/talents, family, group/nationality, character, physical appearance, religion, age, ethnicity, social status, occupation.

Parent homework

Talk to your teen about the news, a TV show, or a moment in history which contains violence. Ask them why they think there is so much violence. Discuss the reactions of the characters and ask what could be done to reduce or prevent the violence. Explain that understanding anger and how you deal with it can help solve the problem. Go over different scenarios of the news, TV show, or moment in history to determine different outcomes. Ask your teen to think of a situation in which they made someone else very angry and what they could have done differently (see Appendix: "Ways to reduce stress").

Maintaining Self-Control: What is Next?!

Nolan was having quite the day. He forgot to set his alarm again. He knew he was going to be in trouble when he got to school. By the time he got to school he had missed his first class. When he signed in at the office the vice-principal told him he was going to have detention after school.

He went to his second class and threw his book on his desk. His teacher was quite upset and yelled at him. His teacher told him he had no right to act that way in her class. She wrote up a behavior slip and had it sent to the office.

For his third class, he had forgotten to do his research paper and it was due today! He told the teacher it was not his fault. He was going to work on it over the weekend but things had come up. His teacher told him he had four weeks to work on the paper and having unexpected events over the past weekend was no excuse for not having the paper ready. His teacher gave him a zero on the paper. Now he was in danger of failing the class.

After class, Nolan fell walking down the steps while on his way to the restroom and hurt his knee. A student he did not know tried to help him up and Nolan started yelling at him. Nolan pushed the student away and told him not to touch him. Just then the student's big brother came down the hall. He was the toughest kid in school. He walked up to Nolan and said no one treats his little brother that way. He was just trying to help. He told Nolan he wanted to see him after school.

By lunch time Nolan was a walking disaster. After he got his lunch he tripped and dropped it on his way to the table; there was food and milk everywhere! That was the last straw, he just could not take this day anymore! Nolan kicked the milk carton across the floor.

One of Nolan's friends came up to him and slapped him on the back and said "How is it going buddy?" Nolan turned around and gave his friend the meanest look and said "Not good! Just leave me alone!" Nolan decided that since everything was going wrong he would just skip school for the rest of the day.

As he was walking off the school property the principal saw him. He had security escort Nolan back into the school. The principal told Nolan that due to the events of the day he was going to be suspended for two days. The principal called Nolan's parents and asked them to come to the school to pick him up.

When Nolan's mother got to the school she was furious! She had to leave work to pick him up and now her boss was angry with her. She told Nolan he was grounded for two weeks. Nolan started arguing with his mother because she knew there was a concert he wanted to go to next week. He had already purchased the tickets. She had to let him go. Nolan's mother told him he was not going to the concert. He started arguing with her more and she extended his grounding to a month.

Discussion questions

- What things did Nolan do that probably made any of the situations worse?

- What could Nolan have done differently to make any of the situations a little bit better?

- Do you think Nolan's friend deserved the greeting he received?

- Do you think Nolan's mother should have extended his grounding? Why?

Steps to keeping self-control

1. Count to ten or higher until you begin to feel yourself calming down.

2. Try to relax.

3. Try to figure out what it is that is really causing you to be upset.

4. Decide what you will do next. Some examples are:

    (a) walk away

    (b) say how you feel

    (c) talk to someone who is not directly involved

    (d) write your feelings down to get them out of your head.

Parent homework

Sometimes you have a day where everything seems to go wrong. The next time your teen has a stressful day, make notes on what was stressing them out and how they reacted. You could make an event/reaction chart. An event/reaction chart would consist of two columns. The first column would list the event that happened. In the second column you would write the reaction from your teen. This way when you sit down to discuss the events with your teen you have notes to help you clearly recall the event and the reaction. When your teen is calmer (hopefully the next day) take the time to sit down and go over what happened the previous day. Talk about different scenarios and how things could have been handled differently. Ask your teen how doing things differently could have improved the situation (or their mood). Feel free to share experiences where you "lost your cool" and talk about how you could have handled things differently to make the situation better.

Avoiding Fights: The Pool Party

It was one of the hottest summers in town for a long time and Justin's parents told him he could have a pool party. He was very excited. He texted all of his friends and told them to be at his house on Saturday at noon. Mikhail said he could stop by for a little while but he had to go to his aunt's house for dinner at 4pm. His parents said they would pick him up at Justin's house since it was on the way.

Mikhail got to Justin's at 1pm. Most of the kids were in the pool but a few were hanging out in the yard and playing games. Mikhail decided to hang with the kids in the yard so he did not ruin his clothes since his parents were picking him up at Justin's. Another one of the kids was getting ready to leave and could not find Justin to say goodbye. Mikhail said he would go find Justin.

Mikhail found Justin in the pool playing volleyball with the other kids at the party. Mikhail tried to yell to Justin but he could not hear him so he swam to the edge of the pool. Mikhail told Justin some people were leaving and wanted to say goodbye. Justin asked Mikhail to help him out of the pool. When Mikhail put out his hand Justin pulled him into the pool. Everyone started laughing. Everyone except Mikhail. He was very angry! He had to leave to go to dinner in an hour and now he was soaked! He had not brought a change of clothes. When Justin climbed out of the pool to tell Mikhail he was just kidding Mikhail pushed Justin and tried to start a fight. Justin told him to chill out. Justin asked Mikhail why he was upset. He had clothes he could borrow to wear to dinner. Mikhail called him a jerk and pushed him again.

Discussion questions

- Why do you think Justin pulled Mikhail into the pool?
- Do you think Justin realized Mikhail would get that angry?
- Do you think Mikhail had the right to be angry?
- Do you think Mikhail handled the situation properly?
- What would you have done if you were Mikhail?

Is this a good way to avoid a fight?

- Someone throws something at you. You pick up something and whip it back at them.
- Someone says you look different today. You yell to them that they look like a freak today.
- Someone starts calling you names. You laugh and walk away.
- Someone tries to start a fight with your friend. You grab your friend and tell them it is not worth it.
- Someone steps on your foot so you kick them in the leg.

Parent homework

Most kids have done something before thinking about the consequences. Think about a time when your teen may have made a bad choice in the spur of the moment. Pick a situation that has not been eating away at your teen. If you pick something that they have been "hearing about" for some time they are going to think you are just bringing it up to hassle them about it again. Ask your teen if they really understand why someone got upset with them. If they are unsure then break it down for them and talk about it until they "get it." It may take time and patience to help your teen understand someone else's point of view especially when they think they did no harm. If your teen just does not seem to understand drop that topic and wait for another opportunity to occur.

Anger Reactions: The Brake Check

Logan was an excellent driver. It took him a few tries to pass the written driving test but he passed the driver's course on the first try. Even his parents complimented him on his driving skills.

One day Logan was driving alone on his way to the mall. There was quite a bit of traffic and it was moving very slowly. Logan told his friends he would meet them at 2pm. There was no way he was going to make it to the mall on time. He started getting frustrated.

Logan finally came to a stretch of road where the traffic was moving at a normal speed. The car behind him passed him and pulled back into the lane in front of him. When the car was in front of him the driver started going very slowly. He was driving under the speed limit. Logan decided to pass him.

After Logan passed him the other driver started following Logan closely. Logan started getting angry. What was up with this guy?! First he passed Logan, then he started driving slowly so Logan passed him, now the guy was riding Logan's bumper! Logan thought to himself "I will teach him a lesson" and hit his brakes abruptly. The driver behind him slammed into the back of Logan's car.

This infuriated Logan! He pulled over and the other car pulled behind him. A witness to the accident also pulled over to see if they could help out in any way. There was quite a bit of damage to both cars. The other driver got out of his car and started yelling at Logan asking him why he slammed on his brakes for no apparent reason? Logan got out of his car and started yelling back at the other driver asking him why he drove like an idiot. The witness got between the two and told them he had called 911 and they could argue over whose fault it was when the police got there. Logan got back into his car and waited for the police to arrive.

When the police arrived both drivers and the witness gave their side of the story. The witness' story sounded the same as the other driver's story. It seemed the accident was Logan's fault. The police officer took everyone's information and told them to resolve their differences in court.

When the court date arrived Logan was charged with reckless driving. His car insurance went up so much that he could not afford to pay for it any longer with the job he had. Logan had to get another job just to pay the insurance premium. Now he had no time to do anything but work. Why did he have to suffer? The accident was not his fault. If the other guy had not driven like a jerk the accident never would have happened. He really hated the other driver for hitting him.

Discussion questions

- Do you think Logan had a right to act the way he did and hit the brakes abruptly?

- Who do you think was at fault for the accident? Why?

- Do you think Logan should have been found guilty of reckless driving?

- Do you think Logan should have to pay more for car insurance?

- What would you have done if you were Logan?

Difference between an anger action and reaction

An anger action is something you do after you have thought through the situation. An anger reaction is something you do before you think.

Is this an anger action or reaction?

- Logan slammed on the brakes for no reason because the car behind him was following too closely.

- Logan took a deep breath and continued to drive normally even though he thought the guy behind him was driving like a jerk.

- Logan pulled over and let the guy behind him pass him and then Logan started following him closely.

- Your favorite hockey team just lost in overtime so you threw your glass of pop at the TV.

- You just stubbed your toe on the coffee table so you kicked the couch and hurt your other foot.

Parent homework

Anger is a difficult emotion to deal with. When we get upset there are usually only two options. We either act or react. For teens going through hormonal changes to begin with it can be increasingly difficult to make an action decision and much easier for them just to react. You cannot be with your teen every minute of the day (and they probably do not want you with them every minute of the day) so it is important to teach your teen the importance of action. Create scenarios that may occur in your teen's life that you know would make them angry. Ask your teen what an action and reaction would be. Then discuss the outcomes of both. It will help your teen realize that if they stop and think and do an anger action the outcome will be much more positive than having an anger reaction. Practice different de-stressing techniques with your teen (see Appendix: "Ways to reduce stress"). The actions will, it is hoped, become ingrained in your teen and they will think before reacting.

Controlling What You Show: The Gift

Ethan's birthday was coming up. He could not wait! Every year his uncle asked him what he wanted and bought it for him. This year Ethan wanted the Cali Flex BMX bike. It was florescent yellow with red rims and black spokes. No one else in his town had one like it. Ethan had pictures of the bike up all over his room. He could not wait to ride it! He told all of his friends he knew his uncle would get it for him.

The day of Ethan's birthday his uncle showed up and said he had a surprise for him but he could not have it until the end of the party. Ethan could hardly control his excitement. Finally it was time for the gifts. After Ethan opened all his gifts his uncle said it was time for his surprise. Ethan's uncle brought in a Cali Power BMX bike. The bike was black with red rims and yellow spokes. It was not the bike Ethan had been looking forward to getting. It was the same make but the colors were different along with the frame design. It was actually more expensive than the Cali Flex but Ethan liked the Flex better. Ethan had researched the bikes for months before his birthday and knew exactly what he wanted. How could his uncle get him the wrong bike?

Ethan was disappointed. Ethan smiled, gave his uncle a hug, told his uncle thank you, and took the bike out for a ride. All of his friends were jealous of his new bike but every time someone said they liked it he told them it was not the bike he wanted.

Discussion questions

- How do you think Ethan felt when he saw the Cali Power BMX bike instead of the bike he really wanted, the Cali Flex?

- Do you think Ethan's uncle knew he was disappointed?

- Why do you think Ethan did not let his uncle know it was not the bike he really wanted?

- What would you do if you were Ethan?

- Would you tell your uncle it was the wrong bike? Why?

Are you controlling what you show?

- You told your friend you wanted to see a particular movie. They bought tickets for a different movie. They apologize and suggest you both see the other movie next weekend. You call them stupid.

- You told your mom you wanted her to pick up toothpaste for you at the store. She buys the wrong kind. She apologizes and says if you do not like it she will get you the right kind. You say it is OK and you try the new toothpaste.

- Your grandmother buys you the ugliest sweater you have ever seen. You put it on to make her happy and tell her you love it.

- Your friend hurt their leg and they have to wear a brace that looks odd. You tell them they look fine and they should not be worried about it.

- You got your schedule for school and you have a teacher you do not like. You walk into class and totally ignore any instructions your teacher gives you.

Parent homework

Sometimes we have to hide the way we really feel to avoid additional problems. If Ethan had told his uncle it was not the right bike both

Ethan and his uncle would have felt bad. Maybe your daughter practiced and practiced for the cheerleading squad but did not make it anyway. Instead of crying she just smiles and says she will try out again next year. Maybe your boss tells you to redo a task that you think is perfectly fine. Instead of arguing with your boss you smile and say OK. Sometimes hiding your true feelings works to your advantage and is more socially acceptable. Ethan was disappointed but showed gratitude. Your daughter was disappointed but showed endurance. You knew it would be better to do what your boss asked instead of arguing the point. Talk to your teen about different situations in which you might have to hide your true emotions. Tell them they can talk about how they really feel with you or a close friend. Hiding the true emotion can ease tension and getting it out to a close friend can validate your teen's feelings.

Chapter **6**

Conflict

Why are we talking about this?

Individuals with ASD sometimes have difficulty understanding conflict. They do not understand why others do the things they may do. If they are faced with a situation that involves conflict sometimes the ASD individual will just shut down. This chapter gives teens the opportunity to discuss various conflict situations safely.

Friends Do Not Get You into Trouble: The Fire

Cameron and Wyatt were sort of friends. They both had groups of friends they usually hung out with and those two groups did not exactly get along. If their friends were unavailable, they would hang out together.

One afternoon when their friends were not around, Cameron and Wyatt decided to go to an old abandoned barn they hung out at. That particular day Cameron had taken matches from the drawer at his house. Wyatt told him he should not mess with matches. Cameron replied "What, are you in kindergarten or something?" and proceeded to light the matches and throw them on the ground.

Wyatt did not want Cameron to tell everyone he was afraid so he lit a few matches himself and threw them on the ground with Cameron. All of a sudden some of the hay outside the barn caught on fire. Cameron and Wyatt tried to put it out but the fire just kept getting bigger and bigger. They both ran away. A neighbor saw the fire and called 911.

The police started questioning all the kids in the neighborhood. One of the boys said that the kids do hang out at the barn but most of them were not there today. Then the police got to Cameron's house. Cameron thought they knew he was there.

When they started questioning him he said he was there with Wyatt. When they asked him how the fire got started he blamed Wyatt. Cameron said Wyatt brought matches from his house and was lighting them near the barn. He said Wyatt was the one who started the fire.

Wyatt had got home a few minutes prior to the police arriving at his house. He was visibly upset. When his parents asked him what was wrong he said he did not want to talk about it and he went to his room. He did not know what he was going to do. Then the police arrived.

The police told Wyatt's parents what Cameron had said. Wyatt's parents called him downstairs to talk to the police. Wyatt was really upset when he found out Cameron had put all the blame on him. They were both playing with the matches. There was no way to tell who actually started the fire.

The police said they were going to open an investigation. Whoever was responsible for the fire would also be responsible for the cleanup fees at the fire site. Wyatt got into a lot of trouble! He was grounded indefinitely.

The next day at school, Cameron saw Wyatt and started laughing at him. He had heard that Wyatt had got into trouble for the fire. Cameron's parents believed that he had nothing to do with it so he was not in any trouble at all!

Discussion questions

- What should Wyatt have done when he saw Cameron playing with the matches?
- Do you think Cameron is going to get into trouble for the fire?
- Was Cameron really a friend to Wyatt?
- Do you think Wyatt should talk to Cameron anymore?
- What would you have done if you were Wyatt?

Is this a true friend?

- A friend stole a ring from a store and asks you to hold it for them.

- A friend tells you not to hang out with someone in the neighborhood who is known for getting into trouble.

- You accidentally hit a parked car and your friend suggests you call the police.

- You accidentally hit a parked car and your friend suggests you drive away and do not tell anyone.

- You see someone drop a credit card and your friend tells you to pick it up and use it.

Parent homework

A lot of the kids shows on TV today touch on social issues. Especially issues with "friends." Peer pressure is everywhere. It could be smoking, drinking, drugs, vandalism, shoplifting, etc. If you are watching a show with your teen in which one of the characters is trying to get another character to do something they know is wrong, point it out to your teen. Ask them what they would do if they were in that situation. If they answer inappropriately ask them why they answered the way they did. If they still do not understand why their answer is inappropriate, explain to them why they are incorrect, what the consequences could be, and explain what the correct action would be (do not do it, tell an adult, walk away, etc.). Kids will get into sticky situations. After all, they are kids. The best we can do as parents is be supportive and help our teens learn from their mistakes.

Apologizing and Accepting the Blame: The Big Mistake

Keisha and Megan were best friends. They spent a lot of time together and even sat next to each other in school. The teacher said they were going to have a math test the next day. Keisha studied for the test but Megan did not. The next day the teacher gave them the math test. Keisha seemed to have an easy time with the test but Megan was struggling. So, she copied Keisha's work. When the teacher was correcting the tests, she realized that both Keisha and Megan had the exact same wrong answers written down.

The next day, the teacher called both girls up to her desk to find out what happened. Both girls denied copying from the other. The teacher said that if one of them did not confess, they would both get zeroes on their test. Megan felt horrible. She did not want her friend to get into trouble for something she did. Megan told the teacher she copied from Keisha. Megan apologized to the teacher and Keisha. She told them both she did it because she did not study and was afraid she would fail the test. She felt horrible. Megan asked the teacher if she could retake the test.

Discussion questions

- How do you think Keisha felt when she was getting blamed for cheating?

- How do you think Megan felt when the teacher said they would *both* get zeroes on the test?

- If Megan did not tell the truth, do you think Keisha would still be friends with her?

- Do you think the teacher should let Megan retake the test?

Are the following kids sincerely sorry?

- "Sorry for getting paint on your pants, but they are ugly anyway."

- "I erased everything on the computer for our class. I guess I pushed the wrong button. I feel really bad."

- "Sorry, I accidently knocked your coffee cup off your desk and it smashed. I will replace it for you."

- "I know I am late for school again but it is not my fault. My mom did not yell loud enough to wake me. It is her problem not mine."

- "I forgot to feed your fish while you were on vacation and it died. But that is OK—we will just get another one."

- "Oh, no—I took the last soda. I did not see you there. Here, we can share."

- "Oh, by the way—I borrowed your bike and left it in the woods. You will find it. Sorry. Bye now!"

- "I dumped iced tea all over your floor. I threw paper towels over it. Someone will clean it up. Sorry."

Parent homework

Sit down with your teen and tell them about a mistake you made which you were sincerely sorry for. Let them know what you did to try to rectify the situation. Explain that no one is perfect and everyone makes mistakes at one time or another. Tell your teen that if they make a mistake and they do not know how to fix it, they can come to you and ask for help. Also, if your teen does make a mistake and apologizes for it, give positive reinforcement, praise them for acting in such a grown-up way, and accept the apology.

Compromise: It is Not Just Another Word in the Dictionary

Jasper's brother was the bass player in a popular band. His brother was coming home from a tour. Jasper asked him if he would give a concert for the locals in their home town. Jasper asked his friend Claire if she would help him with the preparations. Claire happily said yes. She was excited to help out.

There was so much to do! First they found a venue to hold the concert. They could not agree on anything. Jasper wanted to have the concert indoors and Claire wanted it outside. They also needed security. Jasper wanted to call the local police department to see if they would volunteer to do security and Claire wanted to talk to some of her friends to see if they would do it. They needed to advertise the concert and Jasper wanted to hang up fliers but Claire wanted to call the local radio station to see if they could mention something on the air. All they did was argue and nothing was getting done.

Jasper's brother called and said he would be in earlier than expected and asked if they could move the concert date to an earlier date. So far nothing was done and now they had even less time to prepare.

Jasper called Claire and told her the date had been moved. They still could not agree on anything! Jasper said they did not have enough time to argue anymore and Claire should just do what he wanted. Jasper said he was in charge and she was going to do what he wanted her to do. Claire got mad and told him compromise is not just another word in the dictionary. If he was not willing to hear her out he could do it himself.

Discussion questions

- What does the word "compromise" mean to you?
- What do you think Claire meant when she said "compromise is not just another word in the dictionary"?
- Do you think Jasper should listen to Claire's suggestions?
- What would you have done if you were Claire?
- What type of compromises do you think they could have come to?

How can you compromise?

- You are deciding on shirts for your team. You want red and your friend wants blue.
- You are at the beach. You want to swim in the ocean and your friend wants to swim in the pool.
- You and your friend are selling something you purchased together and you are trying to decide on a fair price. You think $100 would be fair and your friend thinks $150 would be fair.
- You are making dinner reservations as a surprise for your parents. You want to go to dinner at 6pm and your sister wants to go to dinner at 8pm.
- You share a room with your brother. He wants to paint the room purple and you want to paint the room blue.

Parent homework

Look up the word "compromise" in the dictionary with your teen. Discuss the definition and ask them what they think it means. Life is full of compromises. Your teen might have to compromise with family or friends on where to go, what to eat, what to buy, etc. Explain to your teen that sometimes they may have to compromise and do something they do not necessarily want to do but the next time they might get what they want. Also explain that flexibility leads to fewer arguments and can work to their advantage in the future.

Rejection: Can She Come to the Movie with Us?

Sloane was quite popular in school. Her parents were well known in the community. She was very pretty and she was head cheerleader. She always got a lot of attention. Sloane was also friendly and had many different friends.

One day she was hanging out with her friend Olivia. Olivia was quite intelligent but she was not very popular. Her parents were not well off and she was a bit plain looking. Sloane was helping Olivia practice for a debate that was coming up in the next few weeks.

The girls from Sloane's cheerleading squad called her and told her they were going to see a movie. It was the movie Sloane had waited for months to get released. She really wanted to go. She had been helping Olivia for a few hours and asked Olivia if she had had enough for the day. Olivia said yes and asked Sloane if she wanted to go to the same movie. Sloane did not want to disappoint anyone so she called her cheerleading friends and asked if they would mind if Olivia tagged along for the movie.

Her cheerleading friends said "What?! You would be seen in public with her? She is not one of us. If you want to come to the movie that is fine but do not bring Olivia." Sloane was crushed. If she did not go to the movie with the cheerleading team she would never hear the end of it. Sloane lied to Olivia and told her she had to go home.

Olivia talked her mother into going to see the movie with her. While they were standing in line she saw Sloane with all the cheerleaders. Sloane saw Olivia in line and tried to hide in her group of friends so Olivia would not see her but it was too late. Olivia's mom asked her why she did not just ask Sloane if she wanted to go to the movie. Olivia told her mother she wanted to go home, stepped out of line, and started walking to the car.

Discussion questions

- Why do you think Sloane did not go to the movie with Olivia?

- What do you think Sloane's cheerleading friends would have said if they saw her at the movie with Olivia instead of them?

- What do you think Sloane's friends would have said if Sloane brought Olivia to the movie anyway?

- How do you think Olivia felt when she saw Sloane at the movies and realized she had lied to her?

- Do you think Sloane was really Olivia's friend?

- What would you have done if you were Sloane and your friends wanted you to exclude someone?

- What would you have done if you were Olivia and you saw that your friend had lied?

How would you deal with this?

- You tried out for a school play but did not get the part you wanted.

- You asked someone on a date and they said no.

- Your friend was invited to a party and did not ask you to come along.

- You went on a job interview and did not get it.

- You applied for a credit card and did not get it.

Parent homework

It is very difficult for a teen to deal with their feelings when they have been rejected. No one likes rejection. Even as adults it is difficult to deal with rejection. It can be a blow to your self-esteem, especially if the person who rejects you is someone you thought was a close friend. Your teen might not freely talk about a time they have been rejected. It is a hard thing to admit to. Tell your teen about a time when you or someone you know was left out of something. Talk in detail about the feelings you felt. Let your teen know it is OK to be upset. Teach your teen socially acceptable ways to accept rejection gracefully. Tell them to talk things out with the person who rejected them to reanalyze the friendship. After a chat they may be able to work things out. If not then that person was not their true friend to begin with. If this happens, be as supportive as you can and remind your teen of the things that make them special, unique, and worthy of true friendship.

Parents Dislike Your Friend: He is Not the Criminal

Zed and Ryan were best friends. They both played billiards, they both rode BMX, they both skateboarded, they liked the same types of movies and TV shows, they had almost everything in common. They even took the same electives in school so they could hang out in class together. Every day after school either Zed was at Ryan's or Ryan was at Zed's.

Zed's parents were not fond of Ryan. Ryan had a brother Will who was always in trouble. Will had recently been arrested for stealing motocross bikes in the neighborhood. He was on house arrest. While on house arrest he decided to go on the run. He would stay at other people's houses so he did not get caught. One day he decided to steal a car and he was caught again by the police. He went back to jail.

Zed could not figure out why his parents hated Ryan. After all, Ryan was not the one who was doing all the illegal stuff. Ryan and Will were exact opposites. Ryan had good grades in school and was never in trouble. After Will got caught stealing the car Zed's parents told him they did not want Ryan at the house anymore and they did not want Zed going to Ryan's house either. Ryan argued with his parents and tried to explain that Ryan was nothing like Will but they did not want to hear it. They insisted that they did not want them hanging out together and said nothing would make them change their minds. Zed's parents told him that if he continued to hang out with Will they would ground him.

Zed was supposed to go to Ryan's house that day after school. Instead he had to call his best friend and tell him his parents would not let him go over. He explained everything to Ryan. Ryan said he understood and he would see Zed in school tomorrow. Zed was very upset. He started yelling at his parents telling them they had no right to tell him who he could and could not hang out with. Ryan was his best friend and he was not the criminal!

Discussion questions

- Do you think Zed should have continued to hang out with Ryan even though his brother was always in trouble?

- Do you think Ryan should have got angry when Zed told him he could not go to his house anymore?

- Do you think Zed's parents had a legitimate reason for telling him he could not go to Ryan's house?

- Do you think Ryan would do the same things Will did?

- What would you do to try to convince your parents to let you hang out with Ryan?

Would you continue to hang out with this person?

- Your best friend just got caught shoplifting.

- Your best friend got a speeding ticket.

- Your best friend assaulted someone because they looked at them in an odd way.

- Your best friend yelled and cursed at his parents.

- Your best friend got into a verbal argument with someone because they called them a name.

Parent homework

As parents we might not like everyone our teens hang around with. There is bound to be at least one friend that you just do not like for some reason. It could be because that friend is always in trouble, maybe they live on the wrong side of town, maybe they come from a bad family, or maybe you have heard some bad things about that person. It is difficult to explain to your teen why you think that person may be a bad influence especially if they are close to that person. We think we know what is best for our teen. Before making decisions try to do a little research. Find out what you can about that friend. What you think you know may be incorrect or you could be right in wanting to be careful. This is one conversation that is going to be difficult no matter how you approach it. When you talk to your teen about an unsavory friend, try not to make accusations. Instead, spend some time alone with your teen and talk to them about the friend. Ask questions about that person. Find out why your teen wants to spend time with that person. If you still feel it is a bad idea for your teen to be around their friend, explain why. When explaining make sure you have your teen's best interests at heart. Do not turn it into an argument. The last thing you want is for your teen to go behind your back to spend time with their friend. If your teen insists that their friend is not a trouble-maker then tell them you would rather their friend spend time at your home. You will feel more comfortable if they are with you and it will give you the chance to get to know their friend better. Maybe they are innocent and there is no better way to find out than to get to know them yourself.

Chapter 7

Family

Why are we talking about this?

Dealing with family situations can be difficult for both the individual with ASD and the family. If there are other siblings in the home without ASD they may find it difficult to understand their sibling with ASD and *vice versa*. This chapter gives both the family and the teen with ASD the opportunity to sit down and talk about various situations that may occur. This will help both the teen and the rest of the family understand each other.

Is This the Right Time? Not Now!

Alyssa is having people over for dinner. Her best friend is coming, her cousins, aunt, uncles, and grandparents. There is going to be a house full of people! Alyssa is cooking three things on the stove, she has a ham in the oven, someone is at the door, and the phone just rang. Her little brother comes into the kitchen and asks her to play a video game. Alyssa gets upset and abruptly says "not now!" Her little brother starts to cry and says she hurt his feelings.

Alyssa feels terrible but she is unable to stop what she is doing to console her little brother. If she does, dinner will be ruined. Why could not he just understand this is not the right time to ask?

Discussion questions

- Why did Alyssa abruptly tell her little brother "not now"?
- Was that the right time to ask Alyssa to play a video game?
- Do you think if her little brother had asked her to play a video game when she was not busy there would have been a different outcome?

Is this the appropriate time?

- You are in line at the department store with your parents. You have waited in line for 15 minutes because the store is *really* busy. Is this the right time to ask your parents to get out of line so you can show them something?
- It is family time at home. Everyone is quietly watching a movie. Is this the right time to call someone on your cell phone?
- Your aunt has come over to teach you how to use the camera you just received as a gift. She is talking about how to take good pictures with your new camera. Is this a good time to ask how to use the flash with your new camera?
- You are outside hanging out with all of your good friends. You do a lot of things together. A new family just moved in next door. The son has come outside and is standing in his front yard right next to where you are hanging out with your friends. Is this a good time to talk about how you are all going to go snowboarding together?

Parent homework

Every parent has encountered one time or another when you were interrupted at the absolute worst time possible. Try to be patient with your teen when this happens. Perhaps create a pin to wear to let your teen know when it is not an appropriate time to interrupt.

Also, make sure you stress that if it is an emergency, *any time* is a good time!

I Do Not Understand My Parents: The Season Pass Dilemma

All Tarin wanted in the whole world was a snowboarding pass at the beginning of the season. In his mind it made perfect sense. The pass cost $300 for unlimited snowboarding during the season. If you paid by the day it was $30 per day. So he calculated that his parents would save a lot of money if they would just buy him the pass. Unfortunately Tarin's parents were unable to afford to pay for the entire pass at this time. They explained to Tarin that he would only be able to go snowboarding once a week and that a season pass just did not fit into their budget right now. Tarin became very angry. He explained the amount of money his parents would save but they just did not understand! Why would they want to pay weekly? It would cost them more money and did they not just tell him they were having money issues? It did not make any sense to him at all! He also explained that he had to go more than once per week. He had different groups of friends and they went snowboarding on different days. How was he supposed to choose who to go with without someone getting mad at him? He went to his room and called his friends and told them his parents were driving him crazy and they just did not understand.

Discussion questions

- How do you think Tarin's parents felt when they had to explain to him that they could not afford the season pass right now?

- Do you think Tarin's friends would be mad at him if he did not go snowboarding with them every week?

- What could Tarin do so he could go snowboarding with all of his friends?

- Do you think Tarin's parents understood how he really felt?

What would you do?

- You buy an outfit that is in style and your parents tell you that you cannot dress like that.

- You listen to music you like and your parents tell you they hate it and to turn it down.

- You dye your hair to show your team spirit and your parents tell you that they will ground you if you do not dye it back to its normal color.

- You want to date someone who is much older than you and your parents say you are absolutely not allowed to date that person.

- Your parents do not want you to go to a party.

Parent homework

We were all teenagers once and I am sure we have all had at least one time where we thought our parents had no clue what we were going through. Being a teen is difficult. Between peer pressure and puberty it is a recipe for mood swings. Remain calm especially when your teen is not. If your teen does not understand your point of view, give them time to think about it. You can also try to explain it in a different way. You can talk to your teen about a time when your parents "just did not understand." It's best to have this conversation when things are calm otherwise your teen may not hear a word you say. There will be times when your teen truly believes you just do not understand what they are going through. When you encounter this do your best to be firm but supportive.

Being an Attentive Listener: Did You Hear Me?

Brian's family was getting ready to go on vacation far away. Brian's mom told him to pack shirts, pants, socks, underwear, shoes, allergy medicine, toothbrush, music player, portable DVD player, DVDs, and his video game for the trip (it was going to be a *long* drive). While his mom was telling Brian what to pack, he was watching TV and just kept saying OK, OK! His mom left the list for him on the coffee table. Brian took the list and ripped it up. He thought he did not need a list.

Brian's mom said they were leaving in five minutes. Brian was still watching TV. Brian went to his room and packed what he thought he might need without asking his mom for help. Then he ran down the steps, got into the car, and they were on their way.

Discussion questions

- Do you think Brian packed *everything* his mother told him to? Why?

- Do you think Brian's mother is going to be upset if he did not pack everything he was supposed to?

- What could Brian have done differently?

Are they really listening to you?

- You are talking to your friend and they answer their cell phone right in the middle of your conversation.

- You are talking to your parents and they ask you questions about what you said because they did not fully understand.

- You are talking to your brother and he is playing a video game.

- You are talking to your sister and she is looking at you and answering questions.

- You are asking your teacher questions and she is offering you help.

Parent homework

Create two or three different totally off-the-wall statements to tell your teen (e.g. "Our house is on skis"). Then say them to your teen at different times of the day (when they are watching TV, playing a game, doing schoolwork, or paying attention). Then later the same day, ask your teen what you told them. See what they can remember (they will probably only remember the one you said when they were paying attention).

Also as parents we expect our kids to listen to us when we talk but we need to remember—when our kids talk to us we also need to listen to them. Take the time to really listen to what your teen says. You will be surprised how much you learn.

Respecting Privacy: You Read My Journal?!

Samantha and her brother Alex were always teasing each other about something. They got into an argument during dinner. Samantha was picking on Alex about Bailey, a girl she knew he liked. She kept teasing him about Bailey. She told Alex that she was going to tell Bailey that he liked her as soon as she saw her tomorrow. Alex was furious! He did not want Samantha to tell Bailey anything! If he wanted Bailey to know he would tell her.

Samantha went out with her friends for a few hours after dinner. Alex decided he was going to get back at Samantha. There had to be someone she liked that he did not know about. He decided to sneak into her room and read her journal. He knew where she hid it because he saw her putting it away one day.

Alex took Samantha's journal back to his room and started reading it. He found out that Samantha had a crush on a boy in her class named Ryan. He decided to keep reading the journal to see if there was anything else he could learn to get back at his sister.

Alex was so into reading the journal that he did not hear Samantha come home. Samantha went into her room and was going to write in her journal when she realized it was gone. She walked into Alex's room and found him reading it. Samantha completely lost her temper. She started yelling at Alex asking him how he could do something like that.

Their parents heard Samantha yelling and came up to Alex's room. Alex's father had a very disappointed look on his face. He asked Alex why he would betray his sister's trust. Alex did not know if he was more upset about Samantha catching him reading the journal or the disappointment he had caused his father.

Discussion questions

- Do you think Samantha really would have told Bailey that Alex likes her or do you think she was just teasing him?

- Do you think it ever crossed Samantha's mind that Alex would read her journal? Why?

- Was it OK for Alex to read Samantha's journal to find out information?

- What would you have done if you were Alex?

- What would you have done if you were Samantha and caught Alex reading your journal?

- How do you think Alex felt when he got caught?

Are you respecting their privacy?

- Your brother has the door to his room shut and you walk in without knocking.

- Your parents have personal documents locked in a safe and you go rummaging through them.

- Your dad leaves his wallet on the table and you do not look through it.

- Your mom leaves her purse in the living room and you look through it.

- Your sister is talking on the phone in her room with the door shut and you are standing outside her door listening to the conversation.

Parent homework

Privacy can be a huge issue with families. It does not have to be between siblings, it could be between you and your teen, your teen and a friend, or even your teen and an employer. It could be something as serious as reading a sibling's journal or something as innocent as snooping for presents but either way it is an invasion of privacy. Talk to your teen about things they may feel are private. Ask them how they would feel if their privacy was violated by a family member or a friend. You want to make sure that your teen understands the gravity of the situation. Something they may see as innocent curiosity could ruin trust between them and someone they care about. It could destroy a friendship or even cause them to lose a job. Make sure when discussing this topic that you do not seem to be accusing your teen of betraying someone's trust.

Sharing Rooms: I Am Not Leaving!

Bailey was hooked on the television show *Rofen High*. It was about a teenage girl's life in high school. Bailey sometimes thought the show mirrored her own life. It was amazing how something could happen to her in school and then she would see it on the show. She never missed it.

Bailey's mom knew how much she looked forward to the show every week. There was a movie on at the same time as *Rofen High* that her parents wanted to watch. Bailey's mom asked her if she would not mind watching the show in her room this week so her parents could watch the movie. Bailey did not mind. It did not matter where she watched the show as long as she did not miss it. Bailey's parents made a point of telling her sister Hannah that Bailey would be watching the show in their room.

Bailey shared a room with her sister Hannah. The difference in their age was only four years but to Bailey it seemed like a ten-year difference. Hannah was in seventh grade and Bailey was in eleventh. They did not share any interests. Bailey thought Hannah was very immature and she really got on her nerves sometimes.

Bailey went to her room to watch *Rofen High*. Hannah was in their room watching a different show. Bailey walked up to Hannah, took the remote, and changed the channel. Hannah started yelling at Bailey saying she had no right to change the channel since she was already watching the other show. Bailey yelled back that mom and dad had told her to watch *Rofen High* in her room and that that was exactly what she was going to do. After all, mom and dad had told Hannah that Bailey would be watching the show and she had every right to change the channel. Hannah argued that she did not want to watch the movie their parents were watching and she hated *Rofen High*. She said the show was stupid and she was there first!

Discussion questions

- Why do you think Bailey thought Hannah should let her watch *Rofen High*?

- Do you think Hannah had a right to be upset when Bailey changed the channel without asking her?

- Do you think Hannah should have been able to watch her show since she was there first?

- What could Bailey have done differently to avoid an argument with Hannah?

- What could Bailey's parents have done to resolve the argument?

How can you solve this problem?

- You are very neat and your brother is not.

- You share a room with your sister and you both wear the same size clothing. She is wearing the shirt you wanted to wear.

- You have bunk beds and you get into an argument about who gets to sleep on the top bunk.

- You like the room warm and your brother likes the room cold.

- You like to sleep with the TV on and your sister likes to sleep with it off.

Parent homework

When teens share rooms with a younger sibling an age difference of a few years can seem like a huge difference to your teen. Even though three or four years does not seem like much the maturity rate of children varies greatly. Arguments are bound to ensue. That is when being a parent seems more like being a referee. It can be hard to be diplomatic when you might ultimately have to choose a side. Even if you have clearly told one of your children about a plan they might still feel slighted in some way. I suggest having a family calendar or family planner. Perhaps make a poster board calendar for each month on which they can indicate in marker if they have certain times they would like to do things. I suggest marker and poster board instead of a white board so things do not accidentally get erased or changed. If it is written in marker it is a bit more permanent and if it is changed it is more obvious. The children can write when they plan on having friends over or when they might need quiet time to study or to do homework. It is a time-consuming project but it can help avoid arguments about scheduling.

Chapter 8

Community

Why are we talking about this?

Individuals with ASD sometimes have a difficult time acclimating to their community. There are various situations a teen can encounter with community activities that they may struggle with. This chapter gives the teen the opportunity to discuss various issues they may encounter in their community.

Safety Concerning Meeting New People: The Dance

Johnna and Cody were both attending the theme dance held at the neighborhood community center. The entire center was decorated with a Hawaiian theme. There were plastic palm trees, grass skirts for the kids to tie around their waist, leis, and even hibiscus barrettes for the girls to place in their hair. [Leis are a Hawaiian custom—necklaces made of hibiscus flowers that are traditionally given to someone to say hello or goodbye. Barrettes help hold the flowers in hair.] They had traditional Hawaiian food and also pizza for those kids who did not want to try something new.

When Johnna arrived she really stood out in the crowd. She was dressed in a beautiful Hawaiian dress and she looked absolutely stunning. Everyone was complimenting her. She felt great that everyone loved her dress.

Then a boy came up to her that she had never seen before. He told her his name was Trevor. She was not sure if he was new to the neighborhood. Trevor seemed like a cool guy so she spent the rest of the dance talking and dancing with him. He got all of her drinks and food for her. All of her friends were jealous because he was talking to her.

Then Trevor asked Johnna if she would like to go for a walk. He said it was too hot in the community center and he wanted to go get some air. He asked her not to mention anything to her friends so they could have time together to talk. She went along with him but did not tell her friends she was leaving. At the end of the dance Johnna's friends were looking for her. Their parents were going to be there soon to pick them up and they could not find her anywhere! They could not even remember the last time they saw her. The only thing they did know was she was dancing with that boy.

Cody was at the same dance as Johnna. He had worked out for weeks getting ready for this dance so he could dress like a surfer. He had on a cool pair of board shorts and even brought a real surfboard with him. A girl walked up to Cody and started talking to him. She said her name was Riley. He had never met her before but she was absolutely beautiful! They talked all night. She was pretty, funny, and they seemed to have a lot in common. Then Riley asked Cody if he would like to go back to her house to watch a movie instead of staying at the dance. She asked him not to tell his friends so they did not give him an attitude about leaving. So he left without telling anyone.

Discussion questions

- Should Johnna have let Trevor get her drinks all night at the dance if she did not know who he was?

- Should Johnna or Cody have left the dance with people they did not know?

- Should Johnna or Cody have left the dance without telling anyone where they were going?

- Why do you think Trevor and Riley asked Johnna and Cody not to tell anyone they were leaving?

Should you trust these people?

- A police officer.

- Someone who walks up to you in a store and asks you to leave with them.

- A firefighter.

- Your parents.

- A neighbor.

Parent homework

Do not let your teen go to any event alone. Make sure they are with a group and there will be adult chaperones. Please sit down with your teen and talk about what they should do if a stranger approaches them or if someone calls them away from their group. Explain that if they have never met someone before they could not even be sure if they are an adult or a peer. You can never be too careful.

General Community Safety: Do Your Parents Know Where You Are?

Decklin thought his parents were the coolest parents anyone could have. They let him do just about anything he wanted to do within reason. All he had to do was let them know where he was and who he was with. It seemed like a fair request so Decklin always let his parents know where he was.

Decklin's parents decided to give Decklin a code word to use if he ever got into a situation that he needed to get out of. If he felt like there could be trouble all he had to do was text the word "blue" to his parents and they would immediately call him and tell him he had to come home. That way, it would not look like he was bailing on his friends on purpose. It was nice to know if something went wrong his parents were there to help him out.

One evening Decklin decided to go driving around with his friends Vince and Darren. Vince had recently gained his driver's license and his parents had let him use the car for the night. Decklin sent a text to his mom letting her know he would be driving around with his friends.

Vince decided to go to the square to hang out. Decklin was not allowed to go there because there was usually trouble going on. Decklin knew his parents trusted him so he decided to tell his parents he was staying at Vince's house so they would not think he was out. He wanted to hang out with his friends and he did not think anything would happen. After all, they were only going to hang out.

When they arrived at the square there were a lot of people they did not know there. Darren decided to hang out with a group of people they did not know. The other group had alcohol so Darren decided to drink with them. Decklin tried to talk him out of it but Darren told him to stay out of it. Darren wound up getting drunk. Darren started a fight with one of the other boys in the group. Decklin and Vince tried to break it up but by that time someone had already called the police. When the police came, Darren got arrested for underage drinking and Decklin and Vince got arrested for disorderly conduct. The police took all three boys to the police station.

The police called all the boys' parents to come and pick them up. They explained over the phone what had happened. Decklin heard the police talking to his mom. He knew he was going to be in trouble when his parents got to the police station. Not only did his parents have to pick him up at the station but also the police had told his mom they picked him up at the square. Decklin knew he was not supposed to be there in the first place and he had not told his parents he was at the square.

Discussion questions

- What was the first mistake Decklin made?
- Do you think Decklin should have told his parents where they were going?
- What could Decklin have done to get himself out of the situation?
- What do you think happened to Decklin when his parents found out?
- Do you think Decklin's parents will ever trust him again?

What should you tell your parents?

- You said you were going to the mall to hang out but your friends decided to go to the movie theater instead.

- You said you would be hanging out with your friend Joe but he went home early and you went to your friend Pat's house.

- Your parents said you could take the car to the mall but all your friends want to go to the park.

- You said you would be at the park playing football but everyone decided to go to get something to eat.

- You said you would be staying over at your friend Danielle's house but Danielle decided you should both stay at Megan's house.

Parent homework

As our teens get older we tend to give them more freedom so they can experience the world for themselves. We trust they will make the right decisions. Unfortunately, teens will make mistakes. One thing they tend to forget is to let you know where they are. It could be disastrous if they are in the wrong place at the wrong time and you have no clue that they are even there. Explain to your teen that they do not need to call you every five minutes to let you know where they are but if they are going to be doing something different from what they had told you they should let you know. Also, giving your teen a code word to use to help them get out of a sticky situation is a good idea. That way if their friends are doing something that makes your teen feel uncomfortable, you can call them and make up an excuse for them to come home. It is always good to give your teen an "out."

Respecting the Property of Others: The Wall

Hector's parents had a small piece of property surrounded by woods that their house was on. They decided to build a rock wall around the perimeter of the property which defined the boundaries of their property. They turned it into a family project. Each weekend they would go for walks in the woods and find stones for the wall. Some of Hector's friends helped out too. They placed each stone by hand. It took them three years to complete the wall and they were very proud of it.

There was a trail through the woods behind Hector's house. A lot of people from the area would walk or bike the trail. It was especially beautiful in the autumn when all the leaves were changing colors. Some of Hector's friends liked to hang out in the woods behind his house. They even decided to put up feeders for some of the animals that lived in the woods. They had bird feeders, corn cobs for the squirrels, and even put up a salt lick for the deer. Every once in a while they would see one of the animals at the feeder. Everyone thought it was cool.

Some of the older kids from school decided to make part of the wall their usual hangout. They would go there after school and sit and talk about their day. Sometimes they would take drinks and food with them. They would leave garbage lying on the ground next to the wall. Hector and his friends found it and decided to clean it up. This became a weekly occurrence. Every weekend when Hector and his friends would walk the trail they would find garbage lying on the ground. After a few weeks of cleaning it up they saw that some of the rocks from the wall had been knocked out of place and part of the wall was beginning to fall down. Hector and his friends decided to fix it.

A few days later Hector had heard about a party that the older kids had decided to have in the woods. He knew exactly who had the party and the kid was known for doing whatever he wanted wherever he wanted. When he went to check out the area there was garbage everywhere and a different part of the wall had been deliberately knocked down. Some of the rocks had been smashed and could not be put back on the wall. Hector was furious! He went home and told his family what he had found.

Discussion questions

- How do you think Hector and his family and friends felt when they finally completed the wall after three years of work?
- Do you think the older kids respected Hector's property?
- What did the older kids do that was disrespectful?
- What would you have done if you were Hector and saw the damage to the wall?

- Is there anything Hector's family could do to prevent more damage being done?

Are you respecting others' property?

- You are on your way to the park. It is shorter to cut through Mrs. Smith's yard. You saw Mrs. Smith planting grass a few days ago. You decide to cut through her yard anyway.

- You are driving down the street and you just finished a drink. Instead of throwing the empty container out of the window you decide to wait until you get home to throw it away.

- You are walking up the street and you see a pile of garbage has blown up against your neighbor's fence. You pick it up and throw it back in the trashcan.

- Your neighbor has boarded up their house for the winter and placed "no trespassing" signs all over the property. You see that one of the doors has blown open. You decide to go into the house and look around.

- A family down the street is known for their prize-winning roses. You see them working on the rosebushes every day. You decided to pick some of the roses for your mother without asking permission from the owners.

Parent homework

As adults we see the line very clearly between respecting and disrespecting someone and their property. For kids the line may be a little blurry. If they are picking flowers for their mother why should that be a bad thing? Most teens think that is a thoughtful gesture. What is the harm in cutting through someone's yard if it is a shorter way to get somewhere? It is not going to hurt anything. It is impossible to cover each and every possible scenario that could occur. Talk to your teen about things they may have done accidentally that led to not respecting someone's property. If you see someone doing something disrespectful point it out to your teen. Ask them why it is disrespectful and ask them what they might do differently. Point out "no trespassing" signs and ask your teen why they might be placed there.

Manners Do Matter: The Dinner

Greyson and Jackson were brothers. Greyson was intelligent and involved with a lot of academic clubs at school. Jackson was athletic and involved with a lot of different sports in school. Their parents, Mr. and Mrs. Aviles, were very thoughtful, caring people who were actively involved in their community. They taught Greyson and Jackson to be respectful toward others even if they were not respectful in return. Their parents told them if someone was disrespectful to them they should be the bigger person and walk away.

One evening their parents decided to hold a community dinner at their home. They were going to invite key members of the community and to try to raise awareness for a community center. They wanted to see if they would have the support of the community to raise funds to build a community center designed with the teenager in mind.

Greyson and Jackson were so excited! Their parents told them they could each invite a friend and their family to the dinner. Greyson decided to invite his best friend from the debate team. They had a lot in common and always had great things to talk about. His friend's family was also influential in the community and Greyson had been to their house on numerous occasions. Jackson decided to invite Owen, one of his friends from the football team. Owen was a great player and recently Jackson had started hanging out with him after practice. Owen was having trouble with one of his classes and Jackson offered to go to his house to help him but Owen said he did not need any help. What Jackson did not know was that when Owen was with other kids he was calling Jackson stuck up. When Jackson invited Owen and his family to the dinner they accepted.

After the guest list was complete there were 10 different families coming to the dinner making a total of 35 people! The Aviles decided to make the dinner a formal affair. They would start the evening with *hors d'oeuvres*, followed by drinks and finally a catered four-course meal. After the dinner they would present their idea for the community center. Both Greyson and Jackson had parts in the presentation. They were going to talk about the lack of things in the community for teens to do and the need for somewhere they could go to hang out and do something fun.

Greyson's friend showed up with his family. They were well dressed and immediately thanked them for the invitation. They knew all of the other families invited to the dinner. They started mingling with the other guests. Owen showed up with his family an hour late. Owen's parents were dressed well but Owen came wearing old, ripped jeans and a stained shirt. He looked like he had not brushed his hair and was quite unkempt. Owen's parents immediately approached the Aviles, apologized for being late and thanked them for the invitation. Owen went to a corner of the room and started talking loudly about other people in the room. He did not have anything nice to say about anyone. Greyson tried to talk to Owen and asked him to relax. Owen told Greyson to get out of his face. By the time dinner came no one wanted to be around Owen. Owen's parents apologized for his behavior. His parents decided it was time to leave before dinner even started. Owen caused a bit of a scene, yelling that everyone there was out of touch with the real world. Then he stormed out of the door. Jackson's parents asked Owen's parents to stay but they apologized for their son's behavior again and promptly left the party.

Discussion questions

- Why do you think Owen did not want Jackson to come to his house to help him with his schoolwork?

- Why do you think Owen and his family were late to the party?

- Do you think Owen's parents were respectful to Jackson's family?

- What would you have done if you were Greyson?

- What would you have done if you were Jackson?

- Would you remain friends with Owen?

Are you being mannerly?

- You are walking down the street and see an older woman in a wheelchair with groceries on her lap. She is struggling to get across the street. You ask her if you could help and push her to the door of her house.

- You are eating dinner in a public restaurant and you burp out loud and then laugh loudly afterwards.

- Your friend buys you a birthday gift. You take it and walk away.

- You are supposed to meet your friends for a 7pm movie and you show up at 7:30pm.

- You are on a bus and there are no empty seats. An elderly gentleman gets on the bus. You stand up and give him your seat.

Parent homework

Manners are something that can make or break your teen. Manners cover everything from polite words, not interrupting someone, behavior while eating to being a good guest. If they are completely disrespectful they can lose friendships. Whenever an opportunity arises point out good manners to your teen, whether it's letting someone in front of you in line because they only have a few items or letting someone pull out in front of you while you are driving in traffic. Explain how thoughtful gestures can improve both your mood and the mood of someone else. Ask your teen how they might feel if someone ignored them or if one of their friends were constantly late for things. Something as simple as saying please and thank you is a way to show respect to people. Modeling good manners for your teen is the best way for them to grasp the concept.

Volunteering: Big Buddies

Greg was required to do some type of community service to meet graduation requirements for his school. They gave him a list of volunteer opportunities. Greg looked over the list and decided to do the Big Buddies program. Big Buddies would place him with a younger boy who was in need of a male role model in his life. Greg was surprised to find out that there was a long waiting list of little buddies in need.

Greg filled out all the paperwork. The application asked a lot of questions about Greg's interests and what he expected to gain from the program. He also had to get clearances to work with children. Greg got a call that they had found the perfect little buddy for him. Greg started to get nervous. What would happen if he did not like the little buddy he was placed with? What would happen if the little buddy did not like him? He talked about his concerns with the program co-ordinator. They assured him they take interests into consideration when pairing up the little buddies with the big buddies.

Greg was placed with a little buddy named Zane. The agency provided Greg with some background information about his little buddy. Zane was eight years old and in second grade. Zane's father had not been actively involved in his life since he was six years old. Zane lived with his mother who worked two jobs. Zane had a stepbrother, stepsister, and two half-brothers he did not get to see. Zane talked about his extended family a lot. Greg was excited when he saw Zane's interest list. Zane loved cars and so did Greg. He immediately started thinking of things he wanted to do with Zane.

The first meeting took place at Zane's home. A representative from Big Buddies was there along with Zane and his mother. When Greg arrived Zane was hiding. His mother talked him into coming into the living room to meet Greg. When Greg saw Zane he instantly liked him. Greg started talking to Zane about cars and Zane's eyes lit up. Greg was amazed when he found out how much Zane knew about cars. Zane was only eight years old and he knew more about cars than most of Greg's friends! When Greg told Zane he had a convertible he ran up to the window to see the car. Zane asked Greg if he could take him for a ride in his car. Zane's mother agreed so Greg took him for a short ride around town. When Zane came back home he had a huge smile on his face.

They set up the first official outing for the following weekend. Greg decided to take Zane to his friend's house. His friend's father collected sports cars and he thought Zane would like to see them. When Greg arrived at Zane's house he was waiting for him on the porch with his mother. He was so excited! Greg took Zane to his friend's house. Zane could not believe the size of the garage! They had a six-bay garage and each bay held two cars. Zane had never met anyone with 12 cars before! He walked around the garage and talked to Greg about each of the cars. He wanted to know everything there was to know about each car. They spent three hours in the garage just talking. Greg's friend told Zane he could pick any car he wanted and they would take him for a ride. Zane picked his favorite and they took him for a long ride.

When Zane got home he could not stop talking about all the things he had done that day. He told his mother all about the cars he had seen and that he even got to pick his favorite and go for a ride! He was happier than she had seen him in a long time. Zane's mother thanked Greg for spending time with him. Greg said he was happy to be with

Zane and could not wait to see him next weekend. There was a huge car show and he had already purchased tickets for himself and Zane. He asked Zane's mother not to tell him because he wanted to surprise him next weekend.

Greg and Zane continued to spend every Saturday afternoon together throughout Greg's senior year. When Greg was ready to graduate he invited Zane to his graduation party. By that time Zane was like part of the family. Zane became very upset when he found out Greg was going away to college. Greg promised to keep in touch with Zane. He called him every weekend and would spend time with Zane when he came in to visit his family. Greg not only got a little buddy, he got a friend for life.

As Zane got older he kept in touch with Greg. They still talked about cars but Zane also went to Greg with things he would go to a big brother about. They were very close. When Zane got to high school he asked his mother if he could volunteer for the Big Buddies program. His mother said yes and told him she was very proud of him.

Discussion questions

- Do you think Greg should have been nervous about the Big Buddies program? Why?
- Why do you think Zane talked about his extended family a lot even though he did not see them?
- Do you think Zane was happy to be paired up with Greg?
- What would you list as your interests in the Big Buddies program?
- Why do you think Zane wanted to volunteer for Big Buddies when he got older?

Finding opportunities:

Research your neighborhood, list your interests, and find different volunteer opportunities that you might like to do. You can create your own volunteer list and maybe even involve some of your friends. Some examples of volunteer opportunities might be:

- helping kids
- getting involved with a political party

- conducting food drives and raising awareness of hunger in the world
- helping preserve parks or places of interest
- helping stray animals
- becoming a driver for the elderly.

Parent homework

Volunteering can enrich your teen's life. They truly can make a difference for someone else if they have the opportunity to do so. Talk to your teen about how they can help others. Ask them how they might feel if someone volunteered to help them, even if it was something as simple as a friend helping them clean their room. Your teen will remember appreciating the help. Help your teen research various volunteer opportunities that match their interests. Get involved with your teen. Help them help others. The feeling you get from helping others and seeing the smile on their face is a huge reward. Make a difference!

Chapter **9**

Relationships

Why are we talking about this?

It seems almost everyone struggles when it comes to relationships in general but for the individual with ASD it is even more difficult. Sometimes it is extremely difficult for them to understand the feelings of their significant other. This chapter gives the teen the opportunity to talk out various relationship problems they may encounter. If the teen is in an active relationship I suggest that after the teen has worked through these stories with someone they also go through them with their partner. It will help both of them understand the other just a little better.

The Bad Reputation: Why is He Going Out with Her?

Keahi just told Becca he is dating Channing, a girl she has heard about. Channing is attractive but Becca has heard a lot of negative things about this girl. Everyone is talking about how Channing smokes, drinks, experiments with drugs, has been arrested, and dates a lot of boys at the same time. Channing does not have a good reputation at all. She is always in trouble with her teachers and her parents. She does not have many friends. Becca asks Keahi what he sees in Channing. Keahi tells Becca that she does not really understand Channing. Keahi's face lights up and he tells Becca that Channing can be sweet, thoughtful, and caring, she is just misunderstood and she is getting a bad rap. Not everything people are saying about her is true. Channing told Keahi that she used to smoke and drink but she never took any drugs. She also explained to him that she was only arrested once and it was not her fault. She was in a car with a friend who had drugs and she got into trouble too.

Keahi tells Becca that if she were really his friend she would be friends with Channing too. Keahi asks Becca to give Channing a chance. He really wants Becca and Channing to become friends so they can all hang out and do things together. Keahi is Becca's best friend and she knows this girl is not good for him. She is only going to hurt him. Why in the world would he want to be with a girl like that? All Becca wants to do is break them up.

Discussion questions

- Do you think everything Becca has heard about Channing is true?

- Do you think Channing is telling Keahi the truth about everything?

- Do you think Keahi really likes Channing? Why?

- Should Becca try to be Channing's friend?

- What do you think will happen if Becca tries to break up Keahi and Channing?

- What can Becca do if she wants to stay friends with Keahi but does not want to be friends with Channing?

What would you do?

- Your friend decides to date someone you know has been arrested for hurting their past boyfriend/girlfriend.

- Your friend decides to date someone you know does drugs.

- Your friend decides to date someone you heard likes to drink but you have never seen drink.

- You have heard rumors that the person your friend is dating is cheating on them.

• Your friend decides to date someone who already has a boyfriend/girlfriend.

Parent homework

It is difficult for kids to understand that sometimes their friends will make relationship decisions they do not agree with. Talk to your teen and explain to them that the decisions their friends make is not a reflection on them. Their friends can make bad choices in relationships but that does not mean they have to stop being friends with them. They can choose not to become involved in their friend's relationship but still be there for them when they need to talk. Tell your teen about a situation you might know of where you had a friend who made it through a bad relationship and how it helped strengthen the relationship you had with them.

Jealousy: But He is My Best Friend

Alden and Brynn had been dating for a few months. Everything seemed to be going perfectly. They enjoyed doing the same things, they were never at a loss for conversation, and they spent every moment they could together. Everyone thought they had the perfect relationship.

Alden's best friend Saul had moved out of town a couple of years ago. Saul's father had received a promotion at work that required them to move. Saul and Alden stayed in touch through email and texts. Alden had told Saul all about Brynn. Saul was coming in for a month over the summer break and Alden could not wait for Saul to meet Brynn. He was sure that Saul was going to like her just as much as he did.

When Saul arrived he spent the first few days spending most of his time with family but did manage to get away to hang out with Alden for a bit. The first day Saul arrived Alden took Brynn to meet him. They did not have much time to chat but he could tell that they liked each other. They made plans to hang out later in the week when things settled down a bit for Saul.

Finally Saul was able to do his own thing. He called Alden and made plans for the weekend. Alden, Saul, and Brynn spent the entire weekend together. They went out to eat, saw a movie, and hung out. They were together all day every day from Friday to Sunday. On Sunday night they were all at the local pizza place and Saul and Alden were making plans for the rest of the week. Even though Saul had only been gone for a year it seemed like it was much longer. So many things had changed in the neighborhood and everyone wanted to see him. Alden said he would get in touch with everyone and make plans for the week.

Brynn liked Saul but she wanted to spend time alone with Alden. They had been going out for a while now and they were always together. She did not mind having Saul around but she missed the times she would have alone with Alden. It seemed Alden did not have much time for her anymore. When she called he would tell her he would call her back because he was making plans. When they did get together it was always Alden, Saul, and other people. Brynn felt like Alden did not have time for her anymore.

Brynn decided to talk to Alden about how she felt. She called him and asked him if he could meet her at the park by himself. He said he would meet her at 6pm. When she got to the park Saul was there too. Brynn pulled Alden aside and asked him why Saul was there when she asked him to come alone. He said they had plans to do something afterwards and he did not think she would mind if Saul were there. After all, they were best friends and anything she had to say she could say in front of Saul.

Brynn got very upset. She told Alden that she hated Saul and she wished he had never come back to town. She said he did not have time for her anymore so she thought they should break up. She left Alden at the park with Saul and went home. Alden apologized to Saul and said he had no idea why Brynn was acting this way.

Discussion questions

- Why do you think Brynn was upset with Alden?
- Do you think Alden was intentionally ignoring Brynn?
- Do you think when Saul went back home things would have gone back to normal with Brynn and Alden?
- What would you have done if you were Alden?
- What would you have done if you were Brynn?

What choice would you make?

- Your best friend asked you to go to a baseball game but your boyfriend/girlfriend hates baseball.

- Your best friend asked you to go shopping but your boyfriend/girlfriend hates to shop.

- Your best friend asked you to go to a party but specifically told you not to bring your boyfriend/girlfriend.

- Your best friend is upset and wants to spend time with you on a night you said you would spend with your boyfriend/girlfriend.

- Your best friend asks you why you are not spending as much time with them since you started dating your boyfriend/girlfriend.

Parent homework

As teens begin to date their social circle may change. When they are exploring a new relationship they want to spend as much time as they can with that person. Sometimes their significant other may have a friend who is always around. This can make a teen feel like they do not have any quality time with their boyfriend/girlfriend.

Talk to your teen about the value of keeping your friends while in a relationship. Boyfriends and girlfriends may come and go but their true friends will always be there for them.

If your teen feels like they are being ignored for their significant other's friends talk to them about how they are feeling. Analyze the situation and discuss whether or not they are truly being ignored or if their boyfriend/girlfriend just likes to be around a group of people. Have them talk to their significant other and possibly set one or two nights a week aside for quality time they can spend together.

Insecurity: The Tutor

Elena and Kyle met at school. Kyle was a basketball player and Elena was a cheerleader. They had a lot of the same classes together. They started talking one day and found they had a lot in common. They even had a lot of the same friends. Kyle decided to ask Elena out and she said yes.

They had been dating for a few weeks. They always went to practice and the games together and then went out with the team afterwards.

Elena was also an excellent student. She was always on the high honor roll and had straight As for the past two marking periods. She would tutor students who were having difficulty in various subjects after school.

A new student transferred to their school named Xander. He was in all the same classes as Elena. Xander was having trouble catching up with his classes. Elena was asked to tutor him in Math and Creative Writing. Elena would tutor him right before practice. So instead of going with Kyle to practice she would meet him there after she was done tutoring Xander. All of Elena's friends were jealous because Xander was quite attractive. Elena's friends started asking her questions about Xander.

Elena told Kyle she was tutoring the new student. He did not really think anything about it until he saw Xander and noticed how all the girls were acting around him. Then all of Kyle's friends told him he better watch out because they thought Xander wanted to date Elena. They told Kyle that since Elena and Xander were spending so much time together it was inevitable that Elena would break up with him. Kyle started getting a little insecure. He asked Elena if she liked Xander and if she wanted to go out with him. Elena tried to explain to Kyle that she was just helping Xander out with his schoolwork but Kyle did not believe her. He accused her of wanting to date Xander. Kyle was upset because she was spending so much time with him. He told her if she did not stop tutoring Xander that he would break up with her. Elena told Kyle that her best friend liked Xander and she was trying to get them together. Kyle still did not believe her. He said she was using it as an excuse to continue to see Xander.

Elena became very upset. She did not understand why he was acting this way. What did she do to make him think she would ever do anything to hurt him? She really cared about Kyle but she did not want him telling her what she could and could not do. She was only tutoring Xander. There was nothing going on between them.

The next day Elena told Xander what was going on. She thought he had a right to know. Xander apologized to Elena for the situation. He said he did not want to cause any problems between her and her boyfriend. He said he would ask for another tutor if it would make it easier for Elena. She thanked him for the offer but she said that she wanted to try to explain things to Kyle one more time. She did not want to date someone who did not trust her. If he insisted that she stop tutoring Xander she would have no choice but to break up with Kyle.

Discussion questions

- Why do you think Kyle felt insecure because of Xander?

- Do you think if Kyle's friends had not said anything he still would have reacted the same way?

- Do you think Elena wanted to break up with Kyle before he accused her of wanting to be with Xander?

- Do you think Kyle had a good reason to be upset?

- What would you do if you were Elena?

- What would you do if you were Kyle?

Are you acting in an insecure way?

- You start to date someone who plays guitar in a band. You go to a show and see them talking to someone. You yell at them and storm out.

- You have been hanging out with someone you have feelings for. They decide to go out on a date with someone else. You call them the next day to see how the date went.

- You are dating someone and they are spending a lot of time with your best friend and asking them personal questions about you. You tell your best friend that if they continue to talk to them you will stop hanging out with them.

- You are out with someone you are dating. They start talking to someone they know. You accuse them of wanting to date that person.

- The person you are dating has remained friends with their ex. You ask their ex to hang out with you and your date sometime.

Parent homework

Teens have a ton of emotions going on at any given time, especially when it comes to dating. If your teen is insecure about anything it can become disastrous for a relationship. If you see your teen going through a time of insecurity talk to them about it. Try to help them understand that what they are feeling has to do with them not someone else. Help them recognize their insecurity and work through it. Share a time when you might have had the same feelings and what the outcome was. Suggest they talk to the person they are dating about their feelings once they understand them themselves. It is to be hoped that it will make their relationship stronger.

Dealing with Differences: The Hockey Game

Tegan and Eric met at the local pizza place one afternoon. Eric was very entertaining and had Tegan laughing all afternoon. He asked her if she wanted to see a movie and she said yes. They made plans for the following weekend.

During the week Eric called Tegan to discuss what movie they should see. He loved horror movies and a new one was just released. It looked really good. When he suggested it to Tegan she said she hated horror movies. She told him they freaked her out and she did not want to see that movie. She suggested a comedy. Eric really wanted to see Tegan so he agreed to go to the comedy movie. He could go to see the horror movie with his friends another time. Eric liked the movie but it was not that great. He asked Tegan if she would like to get together for dinner some time during the week and she agreed.

Eric made reservations at a restaurant in town that he and his family frequented. It was a Thai restaurant and they had fantastic food. When Tegan asked where they were going Eric said it was a surprise. When they got to the restaurant Tegan said that she had been sick from eating Thai food and did not eat it anymore. Eric was disappointed. He told her they could go somewhere else so they went for pizza instead.

There was a hockey game coming up that weekend. Eric's favorite team was in the playoffs and he had tickets right on the ice. He asked Tegan if she wanted to go with him. Tegan was not really into hockey and had never been to a game but she wanted to spend time with Eric so she said yes.

When they got to the game and took their seats they were right up against the glass. Eric was so excited! The game started and it was an intense game. It seemed every time they were fighting over the puck it was right in front of them. Tegan started getting anxious. She did not know hockey could be such a violent game. Then the puck hit the glass right in front of them and it scared her half to death. She jumped and said she did not want to stay for the rest of the game.

The score was tied. Eric did not know what to do. He really wanted to see the end of the game. He started thinking that he really did not have that much in common with Tegan. He asked her what she would like to do if they left. She said she wanted to go to the mall. Eric asked her if she could call one of her friends to pick her up so he could see the rest of the hockey game. Tegan got angry with him and walked out.

Discussion questions

- Do you think Tegan and Eric were a good match to date?

- Do you think Tegan and Eric could be friends?

- Do you think Tegan and Eric had anything in common at all? How could they find out?

- Do you think Eric should have asked Tegan to find a ride from the hockey game so he could see the end?

- What would you have done if you were Tegan?

Can you deal with these differences?

- Your friend wants you to try a food. They love it but you have already tried it and you hate it. Would you argue with them about it?

- You are in a wedding and the bride has chosen a horrible color scheme for the wedding. Would you still be in the wedding?

- You are planning a vacation. You love to fly. Your friend is afraid to fly and refuses to get on a plane. Your friend wants to take a train. It will take six hours to get there by air and two days to get there by train. Do you still take the vacation?

- Your friend loves country music and you like hard rock. You are about to take a road trip. Your friend said since they are driving they should be able to listen to the music they want. Do you go on the trip?

- Your friend likes to bike and you like to skate. Your friend wants to go to a bike park on the weekend. They tell you there are no skateboards allowed but they will bring a bike for you to ride. Do you go?

Parent homework

Some differences are easy to deal with while others are not. Your teen is not going to have everything in common with everyone they meet. Sometimes the differences could be great enough to determine whether or not two people could be in a relationship. Opposites may attract but you need something in common to stay together. Otherwise it could lead to a very stressful relationship. Compromise is great but you should not have to do it all the time. Explain to your teen that sometimes being attracted to someone might not be enough to sustain a relationship. Talk about the other facets of a relationship and how having things in common strengthens it.

Dealing with Rejection: I Wonder Why They Do Not Like Me?

Eva met Nathan at the gym. She had gone there with some of her friends after school. Eva had never been to the gym before so she was having trouble with some of the equipment. Nathan saw her struggling and helped her out. Eva and Nathan immediately hit it off. They started talking about all different things. Nathan asked Eva if she wanted to work out with him at the gym. She said yes so he gave her his gym schedule. They met at the gym four times a week.

Eva and Nathan became very close friends. Eva liked Nathan but she wanted to be more than friends. One day she decided to tell him how she felt. Nathan told Eva he thought she was sweet and she was a great friend but he did not feel the same way about her. He hoped they could still be friends. Eva was disappointed but she said she would still be friends. She went home after the gym that day and felt horrible. Why did she even say anything to Nathan? Would things be weird between them now? She hoped that telling him would not change anything.

Eva saw Nathan at the gym and things seemed normal. They talked just like they did before. Nathan decided to tell Eva about Tess. He had asked Tess out a few months ago but she said no. Then she started dating one of his friends. Now every time he hung out with his friends Tess was there. He told Eva it was killing him to see her all the time after she had rejected him. Eva felt bad for Nathan and told him he was a great guy and anyone would be lucky to be dating him.

Eva went home that day and started thinking about what Nathan had said. She knew Tess and did not know what was so special about her. Tess was pretty but she did not stand out in a crowd. She was quiet and kept to herself most of the time. Tess did not even have many friends. Why would Nathan want to go out with Tess and not her? Eva wondered to herself what was wrong with her? She was pretty. She always had guys asking her out. She had a lot of friends. Why did Nathan not like her the same way she liked him?

The next time Eva saw Nathan at the gym she avoided him. When he tried to talk to her she walked away. When he asked her what was wrong she ignored him. If he did not like her the same way she liked him she just did not want to be around him. Nathan had no idea why she was acting the way she was. The last time they talked everything seemed fine. He called her and left her messages and he also sent her texts asking her what was going on but she would not return any contact. She even changed her schedule at the gym so she did not have to see him there either. Eva thought if he did not want to be with her then she did not want to be around him at all.

Discussion questions

- Do you think Eva should have told Nathan how she felt about him?
- Do you think Nathan understood how Eva felt? Why?
- Do you think Nathan should have told Eva about Tess?
- Do you think Eva should have avoided Nathan?
- Do you think Eva and Nathan could ever be friends again?

What would you say?

- You like someone but they like someone else.
- Your best friend tells you they want to date you.
- You like someone but they tell you they do not like you.
- Someone likes you but you do not like them.

Parent homework

Rejection is hard for anyone to deal with but it's especially hard for teens. They may feel strongly about someone and not have their feelings returned. This could make your teen make some rash decisions such as avoiding the person or ruining a friendship. If your teen is rejected by someone talk to them about their feelings. Talk to them about a time when someone liked them but they did not feel the same way back. Explain that you usually cannot change the way you feel about someone when it comes to dating them. Everyone has different taste when it comes to what they find attractive. You might even want to "people watch" with your teen one day and ask them who they find attractive and who they do not. Ask them if they would date someone they found unattractive. Then ask them if they think the people they did not find attractive are bad people. It will help them understand that just because someone does not find you attractive or they do not want to date you, it is not a reflection on themselves.

Chapter **10**

Cyber Safety

Why are we talking about this?

The internet is a world of its own and individuals with ASD may find it difficult to understand the hidden meaning in instant messages and posts on social networks. Actually, individuals without ASD have a difficult time interpreting things. Cyber safety is very important. This chapter talks about different situations that a teen might encounter while online and gives them the opportunity to discuss the situations.

Video Game Chat: The Cyber Café Meeting

Broden (aka Bro793) was talking online while playing his favorite game, "Island Fortune Hunter." He was getting tips from players all over the world. He was even able to give a few tips of his own. Broden was so proud of himself, especially since he knew some stuff that all those other people playing the game did not know. One of the other members in the room asked Broden if he would do a private chat. He said he wanted to learn more about Broden's tips.

Broden thought it was cool that someone wanted to know more about him so he agreed to the private chat. When they got into the private room Tracker867 started asking Broden all kinds of questions about the game. What character was he? What level was he on? What time did he log on to play? They all seemed like normal questions.

Then things started to change. Tracker867 started asking some personal questions. He wanted to know Bro793's real name. Broden did not think there was anything wrong with that. They had been chatting for a while already so he told him. Tracker867 said his name was Frank. Then Frank started asking Broden all sorts of questions. Where are you from? How old are you? What school do you go to?

Again, Broden thought it was OK to tell Frank the answers to his questions. They had a lot in common and he seemed like a nice guy. Broden asked Frank the same questions. Frank said he was from a nearby town, he was 16 years old, and he went to a nearby school. Frank said "Since we live so close to each other we should meet at a cyber café and play Island Fortune Hunter together."

Broden agreed to meet Frank that weekend. Frank told Broden to tell his parents he was meeting a friend from school so they did not freak out about him meeting someone online. Broden thought that was a good idea because his parents were always giving him a hard time about talking to people he did not really know online.

Discussion questions

- What was the first mistake Broden made?
- What would you do if you were Broden and someone invited you into a private chat?
- Should Broden have told Frank his personal information (real name, where he lived, what school he went to)?
- Do you think Broden should have agreed to meet Frank at the cyber café to play Island Fortune Hunter?
- Do you think Frank was really 16 and just wanted to meet Broden to play Island Fortune Hunter?
- If you were Broden would you have told your parents the truth about who you were meeting?

Should you answer this question in a video game chat?

- Where do you live?
- What school do you go to?

- Where do you hang out?

- Are you ever home alone?

- Do you enjoy playing the game?

Parent homework

Online gaming is becoming increasingly popular among teenagers. With the current game systems all you need is a phone line and a subscription and you can play your video games with people all over the world. This poses a whole new safety issue. Make sure you talk to your kids about the people they are talking to online. Maybe even ask them if you can watch them play their video game and make a mental note of the other people they are talking to. Explain to your teen how dangerous it could be to meet someone you have met online without knowing who they are. Listen to your teen when they talk about who they are playing games with online and ask questions about the other players. If you ask questions maybe your teen will too.

Social Networking Sites Event Invitations: I Know When Your Party is

Brandon was turning 16 and decided to have his birthday party at his house. He had an in-ground pool and a large yard so it would be perfect. His parents told him since it was his sixteenth birthday he could invite as many people as he wanted. Brandon wanted his party to be huge so he decided to invite everyone he knew.

Brandon started writing out invitations to the party and after looking up addresses and addressing the envelopes he got impatient. He thought there must be an easier way to do this. He decided to take a break and go onto Bamboo Frame and check out what his friends were doing and maybe play a game or two.

Bamboo Frame was a social networking site that one of his friends had told him about and that he had been on for about a year. In the beginning he only had a few friends. As time passed more and more of his friends joined. As he started playing the games he got more and more friend requests. Most were from people he did not know. At first he did not approve the requests but after a while he just started approving everyone and did not really check to see who they were. If he got multiple friend requests he would just "approve all." What harm could it do? Now he had over 700 friends from all over the world!

While he was on Bamboo Frame his friend Hannah instant messaged him. Brandon told her about the party and told her what a pain it was to write out all the invitations. Hannah suggested he post it on Bamboo Frame Events and invite his friends that way. Brandon thought that was a great idea! He would not have to write anymore and everyone he knew was on the site anyway. It would be so much easier!

Brandon went on to the events page and made up a posting. He included his address and the day and time of the party. All he had to do now was go through his friends list and pick who he wanted to invite. He started paging through his friends list and checking the boxes for who he wanted to invite. This started to become time consuming too. So, instead of individually checking the boxes he just selected "check all." He thought it would be a lot quicker and he knew that if someone lived in a different country they would not be able to come anyway.

What Brandon did not realize was that Tevin was still on his friends list. They knew each other but Brandon had found out that Tevin was trouble and did not talk to him anymore. Tevin also got an invitation to Brandon's party.

Tevin really did not like Brandon. He thought Brandon thought he was too good to hang around with Tevin and his friends. Brandon never did anything with Tevin's group and Tevin heard that Brandon was saying bad things about him.

Tevin decided he would talk to some of his friends and go to Brandon's party and try to cause trouble. He wanted to pay back Brandon for all the things he heard he had said about him.

Discussion questions

- Should you approve everyone that sends you a friend request? Why?

- Was it a good idea for Brandon to create an events posting on Bamboo Frame?

- Should Brandon have done the "check all" for the invitation to the event?

- How do you think Brandon felt when Tevin and his friends started causing problems at the party?

- How do you think Brandon's parents felt when the trouble started at the party?

Should you post these things on a social networking site?

- You decide to skip school and post it on the site.

- Your complete home address.

- Your cell phone number.

- When you and your family are going to be out of town.

- Your email address.

Parent homework

Social networking is a way of life. Kids are on many different sites and they might approve friends who they do not know. Event scheduling is a convenient way to let everyone know when something is happening. Using the social networking site to invite people to events has become commonplace. Explain to your teen that they might inadvertently give out personal information to people they do not want to have it. Encourage your teen to take the time to sort through their friends list and only include the friends they really want to attend the event. It may take time but it can avoid potential problems and it is still faster than mailing invitations. Also, employers have begun to use social networking sites to check up on potential employees. Tell your teen to be extra careful what they post and to make sure permissions are set so only people they know can see their information and posts. It could make the difference in getting a job.

Cyber Bullying: I Will Get Them!

Nicholas and Bella were twins. They both did well in school but neither one of them was very popular. They kept to themselves in school and sat together during lunch. Sometimes the other kids would make fun of the way they dressed or how they spent so much time together. They would also call them "teacher's pet" because they did well in their classes and the teachers always complimented them on their thoughtful answers and their participation in class. One girl in particular, Caite, was ruthless. She was always making fun of Nicholas and Bella.

Finally one day Bella had had enough. On the way home from school she was talking with Nicholas and said she just could not take it anymore. She had to figure out a way to get back at Caite. Nicholas suggested creating a website that made fun of Caite. They were not the only ones that Caite made fun of. They could blog the site name to everyone in school. Then everyone would have the opportunity to make fun of Caite the way she made fun of them.

Nicholas was a wizard at creating websites. He had the site up and running in a matter of hours. He named it WeHateCaite.com. He blogged the name of the site to everyone in school. Within days there were pages and pages of insulting comments about Caite. They made fun of her. They also posted how mean and hurtful she was. Even her friends posted nasty things about her.

Caite found out about the website from a friend. At first when she went on the site she thought it was a joke. Who cares what these losers thought of her? Then she saw the comments posted by her friends.

Discussion questions

- Why do you think Caite was so mean to Nicholas and Bella?

- Do you think Nicholas and Bella should have created the website?

- What would you have done if you were Bella?

- What would you have done if you were Nicholas?

- What other ways could Nicholas and Bella have dealt with Caite's teasing?

- How do you think Caite felt when she saw the comments posted by her friends?

Is this cyber bullying?

- You heard a nasty rumor about someone at school and you post it on a social networking site.

- You post mean comments about someone on your blog.

- You threaten someone through instant messaging.

- You harass someone through email.

- You post someone's cell phone number on a daily feed.

Parent homework

Things are significantly different from when we were kids. The information technology available today is astounding. Kids have many different outlets to bully other teens such as texting, blogging, posting comments, posting pictures, creating websites, etc. Many teens have become cyber victims of bullying. There can be legal ramifications with cyber bullying. There have even been reports of teen suicide due to cyber bullying.

Ask your teen if they know of anyone who has experienced anything like this. Ask them how that person felt when they found out. Talk to them about how they would feel if someone did it to them. If your teen becomes a victim discuss various solutions to both bullying and cyber bullying. Let your teen know they are not alone. There are different solutions other than revenge. Teens can be extremely hurtful and you need to let your teen know they are not alone. Help them rebuild their self-esteem and help them realize who their true friends are.

Social Networking Status Updates: How Did They Find Us?

Mitchell and Kiera were hooked on Utell. It was a status updating program for their phone that would post their status to anyone who subscribed to the feed. They were always posting stuff on Utell. They both posted when they woke up, when they got to school, how school was going, what they were doing afterwards, and where they were at all times. All of their friends subscribed to their feeds so they could meet up. Kiera was very careful who she accepted to subscribe to her feed but Mitchell never really paid attention to who was subscribing to his feed. He just approved everybody. He thought the more people around the more fun it could be.

When Kiera broke up with her boyfriend the first thing she did was delete him from her Utell feed. Kiera had liked Mitchell for a while. After she broke up with her boyfriend she started posting about it on Utell for a couple of weeks. All her friends knew how she felt about him. Finally Kiera decided to see if Mitchell would go to the game with her at the weekend.

Kiera decided to subscribe to Mitchell's feed so he subscribed back to hers. She asked him to go to the game with her on Friday through Utell. He replied yes. Then he read her other posts and found out that Kiera had just broken up with her boyfriend. He also saw the posts she had made about him. He was happy to see she felt the same way about him as he did about her. Mitchell decided to post how he felt about Kiera on Utell. He posted that he had liked Kiera since the first time they met.

Mitchell's friends told him that Kiera's ex-boyfriend was going to be at the game with all of his friends. They heard that Kiera's ex-boyfriend was upset about the break-up and that he thought she broke up with him to go out with Mitchell. Mitchell did not want to back out on the date so he called Kiera and asked her if she would like to go somewhere else. She thought it would be a good idea. So they made plans to go to a movie.

The night of the movie both Kiera and Mitchell posted where they would be. They thought some of their friends could meet up with them after the game. When they walked out of the movie they saw Kiera's ex-boyfriend and all of his friends waiting for them. How did they find out? Mitchell asked Kiera if she had told him. She denied it and said she even deleted him from her Utell feed so he would not know what she was doing. Mitchell checked on the people subscribing to his feed and found out that Kiera's ex-boyfriend had sent a request to him a few weeks ago and he had accepted it without realizing it. Kiera's ex-boyfriend knew what was going on since he subscribed. He had received all of Mitchell's posts including the one that said they were going to a movie instead of the game. He even posted what movie and what time they would be out in case anyone wanted to meet them afterwards. He did not expect to see her ex-boyfriend there.

Luckily security for the movie was in the lobby and noticed the group of people. The security guard walked over to Kiera and Mitchell and asked them what was going on. Kiera explained to the security guard what had happened. The security guard walked them to their car. As soon as they got to the car Mitchell deleted Kiera's ex-boyfriend from his feed and posted to his friends what had just happened and that they were going to the coffee shop next. His friends replied to say that they would meet them at the coffee shop.

Discussion questions

- Should Mitchell have accepted everyone who requested to be part of his feed on Utell?
- Why do you think Kiera's ex-boyfriend thought she had broken up with him to go out with Mitchell?
- Do you think Mitchell should have gone through everyone he had accepted and deleted them if they were not a good friend of his?
- Do you think Mitchell should have posted where they were going after the incident at the movie theater?
- Do you think Kiera's ex-boyfriend was able to find out they had gone to the coffee shop? Why?

What would you accept or post?

- Would you accept a feed request from someone you do not know at all?
- Would you accept a feed request from someone you do not know very well?
- Would you accept a feed request from a friend?
- Would you post where you are every minute of the day?
- Would you post personal information such as your home address or cell phone number?

Parent homework

With all of the technology today someone may completely lose their privacy and not even know it! Kids like to post things on social networks. They think it's fun to put up everything that is going on. The problem is they might not know who is reading it. Even if they do not accept everyone to their feed, someone they do not want to communicate with might know someone who is subscribed to the feed. Teens really need to be careful who they allow to follow their status updates. If someone asks to subscribe and your teen does not know who it is or they feel the person's character might be questionable tell them it is best to not accept them. It could avoid many problems in the future. Also, letting people know when you are not going to be home or when your parents are not going to be home could result in a safety issue. Advise your teen to be very careful what they post.

Social Networking Sites Posting Pictures: Why Are My Parents So Upset?

Callie and her friends were always on Piks. Piks was a social networking site that let you post photos of yourself and your friends. You could tag a photo if your friend was in it and it would show up on their profile. Every time Callie and her friends went somewhere they were taking photos and posting them from their cell phones. Callie's profile had over 200 photos that her friends tagged her in. Those did not include the photos Callie had posted herself. She had over 500 photos on her profile!

There were privacy settings on Piks. Callie let everyone see all her photos. She did not see the point of limiting who saw her photos. The point of putting them on the site was so everyone could see them.

One of Callie's friends decided to have a party while her parents were out of town. Callie told her parents she was staying at her friend's house but she did not tell them about the party. A girl named Nadya was at the party and she did not like Callie. Nadya decided to post photos from the party on Piks. Callie was in a lot of the photos Nadya posted. She usually checked when she was tagged in a photo but she had to leave early the next day to go to dinner with her parents so she did not get a chance to see what Nadya had posted. After dinner Callie went back to her friend's house.

While Callie was at her friend's house her parents got a phone call. One of her mother's friends was looking at the Piks site and came across Callie's profile. Some of the photos from the party were up. Her mother's friend told her parents about the photos. Callie's parents logged on to Piks and looked at the photos.

Callie's parents called her at her friend's house and asked her what they had done the night before. Callie had told them that some people had stayed over at her friend's house but she still did not tell them about the party. Her parents told her they had seen photos of the party on Piks and wanted Callie to come home immediately.

Callie's parents were very angry. They were upset that Callie had not told them about the party. As soon as she got home Callie's parents went on the Piks site with Callie. When Callie saw some of the photos she got really upset. Nadya had pictures of her posing in her swimsuit and the pictures looked a little inappropriate. Nadya had also tagged Callie in photos she was not even in. There were lots of photos of people drinking at the party. She had tagged Callie in the photos so they were posted on her profile! Then Callie's parents decided to go through all of Callie's photos. They had never gone through them before because they had trusted her daughter. They were not pleased with what they found.

Callie knew Nadya did not like her but she never thought she would do something like this. Callie tried to explain but her parents did not want to listen. Her parents told her they were very disappointed in her. Callie's parents made her delete her profile on Piks and she was grounded for the rest of the semester. Callie was very upset about deleting her profile. There were some photos on the site that she did not have saved anywhere else and now they would be gone forever.

Discussion questions

- Why do you think Nadya tagged Callie in the photos even if she was not in them?

- Why do you think Callie had posted photos of herself that might make her mother upset?

- Do you think Callie wanted to disappoint her mother?

- Should Callie have set privacy settings on her account?

- Do you think Callie's mother should have made her delete her account?

Would you post or tag these photos?

- Would you post a photo of your house with the house number clearly visible?

- Would you post photos of yourself and your friends out somewhere when you are supposed to be at work?

- Would you tag funny photos of people you work with but not tell them you are posting them?

- Would you post and tag photos of your friends and family?

- Would you tag photos of people if they were not in the photo? Why?

Parent homework

If your teen is part of a social networking site there is a good chance they have photos posted. You might want to talk to your teen about their privacy settings on their account. Also talk to them about what may not be appropriate to post. There are many teens out there that post provocative photos but they do not think they are. Sit down with your teen and look at some of the photos they have posted and the photos their friends have posted. If you find some inappropriate photos talk to your teen about them. Ask them if they think they are inappropriate. You could also create a profile yourself and become a friend to your teen on the site so you could see the content. It can be fun to see both your teen's and their friends' photos.

11

Classroom Skills

Why are we talking about this?

Individuals with ASD sometimes also have attention deficit hyperactivity disorder (ADHD) or obsessive compulsive disorder (OCD) along with their ASD. This chapter talks about how to deal with different classroom situations where ASD or these other disorders may affect their performance in the classroom.

Paying Attention to the Task: Anything but Schoolwork

Chris absolutely hated History class. Not only was he not interested in history but the teacher was so boring! The teacher talked in a monotone voice and Chris just could not pay attention no matter how hard he tried.

Chris was a sociable student so every day he walked into History class he would chat with his classmates. It did not matter who it was, he would strike up a conversation about anything but history. He would talk about what they did the night before, football, baseball, biking, skateboarding, a new movie, the weather or anything else that popped into his head as long as it had nothing to do with history.

After class started Chris would stare out of the window and think about what he was going to do when he got out of school. If it was nice out he thought about what he would do outside, if it was raining he started thinking about video games or whose house he was going to. He did not pay attention to anything the teacher had to say.

If the teacher asked him to pay attention he would look at the teacher but his mind still was not on the class. He would start tapping his pencil on the desk or start drawing on a paper. Sometimes he would try to strike up a conversation with one of his classmates again or he would pass notes. He never took notes in class.

When midterm reports rolled around Chris was excited. His parents told him if he passed all his classes they would take him and two of his friends to the beach for the weekend. He could not wait! He had already asked his two best friends to go. They had been making plans for the past month. There were so many cool things to do at the beach.

When Chris received his midterm report he was devastated. He was failing History class. The trip to the beach would be cancelled. Now he had to tell his friends that the weekend they were looking forward to would not happen. He knew his parents and his friends would be disappointed. Chris thought he could explain it to his parents. After all, it was not his fault. If the teacher was not so boring he would be passing the class.

Discussion questions

- Why do you think Chris was failing History class?
- How do you think Chris' friends felt when they found out the trip might be cancelled?
- Do you think it was the teacher's fault Chris was not passing?
- Do you think Chris' parents believed him when he said it was not his fault?
- What could Chris have done to improve his grade in History class?

Are these students paying attention?

- A student is looking out of the window.
- A student is drawing in their notebook.
- A student is taking notes.

- A student is doing the assignment on the board.

- A student is passing notes when the teacher is talking.

Parent homework

I think at one time or another we have all had a teacher that we just did not click with. Personality conflicts with your teacher can make it hard to concentrate in class. Explain to your teen that sometimes they will get a teacher who just does not fit their learning style. If this happens talk to your teen about different ways they might be able to improve in the class such as talking to the teacher and asking for extra credit. Help your teen in any way you can to get them through that class with a passing grade. Explain to your teen that if they pass the class they will not have to take it again and it is to be hoped they will not get that teacher again. If they do, work out a plan to help your teen be successful in the class.

Following Specific Instructions: The Kilter System

Gage was saving his allowance for months to purchase the new Kilter System. It was the latest and greatest in game systems. It had a free online gaming service and it also had a movie library from which he could stream movies directly to his TV. He finally had enough money and his father took him to the electronics store to buy it.

Gage's father told him he would help him set up the system but he got called into work that evening. Gage could not wait. He wanted the system hooked up now so he decided to try to set it up himself. The Kilter System was advertised as the easiest game system to set up. He glanced at the directions. For an easy system to set up there were quite a few directions. Instead of reading the directions he just glanced at the diagram. It seemed that all he had to do was connect the system to the TV and it would work.

Gage plugged the wires into the game system and connected the wires to the TV. Then he plugged in the game system and turned it on. The power light came on the Kilter System so he inserted the game which came with the system. He turned the TV on and waited for the game to come up on the screen. The TV screen stayed dark. He turned the system on and off a couple of times and still nothing. Gage became more and more impatient. He turned the TV on and off and he made sure everything was plugged in where it was supposed to be.

After trying everything he could think of he gave up. Gage called his father at work and told him that the Kilter System must be faulty and they would have to return it to the store for a new one tomorrow. Gage's father told him he would look at it when he got home from work. Gage knew he would have to wait until the next day to use the system, if it even worked, since his father did not get home until very late in the evening.

Gage's father immediately went to Gage's room as soon as he got home from work. He knew how much Gage was looking forward to getting the Kilter System set up. He wanted to surprise Gage in the morning by having the system set up and working for him when he woke up.

Gage's father looked at the diagram and checked it against what Gage had completed. It all looked correct. Everything was plugged into the right spot and there was power going to the system. His father turned on the TV and there was a blank screen. Gage's father read over the detailed directions and it clearly stated that the TV had to be on Channel 15 in order for the game system to work. His father checked the channel and Gage had the channel on 11. As soon as Gage's father changed the channel to 15 the game system worked. His father turned the channel back to 11 and went to bed.

Discussion questions

- What was the first mistake Gage made?

- What were the consequences of Gage not following the specific directions?

- Why do you think Gage's father turned the channel back to 11 instead of leaving it on the correct channel?

- What do you think happened when Gage woke up in the morning?

- Do you think Gage went back and actually read the directions?

- How do you think Gage felt when he realized there was nothing wrong with the game system?

Should you follow specific directions?

- You just got a new cell phone and are having trouble figuring it out.
- You are trying to put a bookcase together.
- You are doing a homework assignment.
- You are playing a new game.
- You are driving to a destination you have never been to before.

Parent homework

Many things we encounter require us to follow specific directions. Some parents still shudder at the words "some assembly required." I think most of us have tried to shortcut reading all the directions and trying to put something together in a hurry only to have to take the entire thing apart and start from the beginning. Talk to your teen about a time when you tried to rush through something and missed a step. Talk about your frustration; let your teen know they are not the only person in the world who might do this and feel this way. Explain the importance of following the specific instructions from the beginning. Sometimes even if you follow the instructions to the best of your ability you still might make a mistake. I cannot tell you how many times I have put something together only to realize half way though that I had put the wrong pieces in place because I did not look at the labels. Putting together a toy or a model with your teen is an excellent way to teach the importance of following specific instructions. Find something you and your teen would enjoy and have fun putting it together.

Completing Assignments on Time: The Research Report

Jaimsie had a research report to do for her English class. The teacher worked with the students on picking a topic and setting up an outline. The students had a month to complete the paper. It had to be ten pages long and they needed to list at least five different references.

Jaimsie chose to write a report on medieval lore. She had been fascinated with castles, dragons, and knights for as long as she could remember and thought that would be a perfect topic for her report.

Since she already had the outline done she was not in a hurry to start the report. After all, how hard could it be to put the report together if she already had the outline? She already knew a lot about the topic and had many books about medieval lore. This research report would be easy to complete.

The weeks went by quickly. Jaimsie had plans to do things with her friends almost every day. She was always busy doing something. Her friend called her one evening and asked her if she was ready to turn in her research report. Jaimsie told her friend she had not even started the report yet. Her friend told her she had better get to work since the report was due the next day! Her friend had the due date on her calendar at home.

Jaimsie went into a panic. There was no way she was going to get a ten-page report done in a few hours. She thought her teacher was going to be so upset with her. She would be embarrassed in front of the entire class when she did not have a paper to turn in. She was going to get a failing grade for not doing the research paper. What was she going to do? Jaimsie started thinking up excuses to tell the teacher why the report was not done.

Discussion questions

- What was the first mistake Jaimsie made?

- What things could Jaimsie have done to make sure she got the report done on time?

- Do you think Jaimsie should have made up excuses to tell her teacher or do you think she should tell her teacher the truth? Why?

- Is there anything Jaimsie could have said to her teacher which would mean not getting a failing grade on the report?

What would happen if…

- You turned in your homework on time.

- You turned in your homework a day late.

- You turned in your homework a week late.

- You turned in your homework a month late.

- You never turned in your homework.

Parent homework

Deadlines can be stressful especially if you forget about them. Some teens tend to procrastinate when it comes to assignments that seem daunting. Teens could have numerous deadlines for various different classes all happening around the same time. If your teen does not have a system it is quite easy to forget about something. Talk to your teen about deadlines and due dates. Tell them about a time when you missed an appointment or a deadline. Tell them how you felt and what consequences you had to face. Work up some type of system, possibly a calendar, so your teen can see the due dates for various assignments. Talk to your teen about the importance of doing a little bit each day instead of facing a colossal task the night before it is due. If your teen develops these habits early it will make school a lot easier in the future.

Doing it Right the First Time: The Rush Job

Mia was always in a rush to get her work done. It did not matter what class it was or what the assignment was, she always wanted to be the first one done with the assignment. As soon as the teacher started giving directions Mia would start to work. She never heard all of the directions. When she finished the assignment it was never completely done. Mia's teacher told her to "slow down, take your time, and look over the directions" but Mia just kept speeding through her work.

She would almost always be the first to hand in the assignment. Her teachers would tell her to go back to her desk and look it over. Mia did not need to look it over. She was already done with the assignment, what else was there to look at? Mia did not want to disrupt the class when she was done with her work. She would go back to her desk and begin to draw or talk softly to a peer who was also done with their work.

Discussion questions

- Why do you think Mia always wanted to be the first one done with the assignment?

- Do you think her friends were impressed because she was always the first one done with the assignment?

- Do you think Mia had to do a lot of assignments over again?

- How do you think Mia's grades were in her classes?

Scenarios

Look at the following scenarios and decide whether or not the job was done right the first time. If it was not done right the first time, how could the student fix the work?

- John was the first one done but no one could read his work because he wrote too fast.

- Mary finished her math homework but all of the answers were wrong because she just put down any number to make it look like she was done.

- After reading the directions Larry completed his reading assignment. The directions said to write down the words that have the same meaning. Larry wrote the words that mean the same.

- Ben wrote a book report on the computer. He listened and followed directions when his teacher told him to save his work frequently. The computer crashed. Do you think Ben had to redo all his work?

Parent homework

Some teachers give students the opportunity to fix their mistakes but some teachers do not. It is important for your teen to learn to do the job correctly the first time. If they do they will not lose time having to redo the assignment and they will also get a better grade. Try to get your teen into the habit of looking over their homework after they are done. This will, it is hoped, transfer into the classroom and they will begin to look over their assignments carefully when they are complete. It does not do a student any good to rush through an assignment. All the kids have the same amount of time to complete an assignment and there is no glory in always being the first one done. If your teen uses their time wisely in the classroom they will greatly benefit from it.

Test Anxiety: I Knew it Yesterday!

Addison had a college entrance exam coming up. This test was extremely important. Addison knew which colleges she wanted to apply to and she had to do well on the entrance exam or she would not even be considered for admission.

Addison had had problems taking tests before. Her teachers would make accommodations for her in school. She did not know if she would be able to get accommodations for the entrance exam so she decided to take a course on the entrance exam. Every weekend for two months she went to a class that went over various parts of the test. It gave sample questions and test strategies on how to answer different types of questions. The course did not cover how to deal with the anxiety of the test. Addison felt like she was ready to take the exam. She scheduled it for two weeks later.

Addison studied every night for those two weeks. She knew the exam was going to be difficult but she felt confident that she would pass with a good score. If she did not get the needed score she could not take the exam again for six months. That would mean she would not be able to start college that fall and she would have to wait for the spring semester. She wanted to start on time. She already had her classes planned out and knew when she wanted to graduate. She had put a lot of thought into this and it was all riding on her getting the score she needed.

Addison had made up her own practice tests. She knew what kinds of questions were going to be on the test. She continually went over and over the material. Her parents quizzed her on the material the night before the test and she had all the answers right. She was confident that she would do well on the exam.

Addison tried to go to bed but she could not sleep. She just could not get the test out of her head. She just had to do well or everything would be ruined. She tried to talk to her parents about it but they just told her that if she did not get the needed score this time she could always retake the test. They just did not understand how important this was to her.

The morning of the exam came and Addison was so nervous she did not even eat breakfast. Her stomach was killing her but she went to the test site anyway. When she sat down she started getting dizzy. The administrator passed out the test and told them they could begin. Addison opened the test booklet and started reading the first question. She did not understand it at all. She knew she had studied the material and she even remembered going over a question like this one but she could not remember what the answer was. She started feeling sick. Addison knew she could not leave the room and come back to the test. She went on to read the next question. The same thing happened. It was like the test was written in a foreign language. She did not understand any of it! Why could she not just remember the answers? She knew them yesterday!

Addison remembered a technique one of her teachers had taught her. It had helped her with some tests in school when she had got nervous. Addison took a deep breath, closed her eyes, and tried to relax. Then she started the test over again.

Discussion questions

- Should Addison have called the test administrator to find out if she could get accommodations for the test?

- Do you think Addison could have done anything else to prepare for the test?

- Do you think Addison's parents understood how important the test was to her?

- What would you do if you were Addison and felt sick during the test?

- What did Addison do right?

- How do you think Addison did on the test? Why?

Are you feeling test anxiety?

- You can't sleep the night before an exam.

- You eat a healthy breakfast the morning of the exam.

- Your stomach starts to hurt the moment you set foot in the classroom.

- You are having a hard time remembering the answers so you close your eyes, relax, and start the test over.

- You can't sit still while you are waiting to take the test. You are tapping your foot, bouncing your leg, and chewing on your pencil.

Parent homework

Test anxiety is horrible! It can manifest in many different ways. You may think your teen is just trying to get out of taking a test but their anxiety may actually be causing them to get ill. There are various techniques to help them get through the test anxiety. Relaxation techniques such as deep breathing work well. Sometimes exercise before a test can help reduce some of the anxiety. If allowed, chewing gum, having some type of hard candy, or just taking a drink of water can relax a student. Also, teaching your teen testing strategies can reduce some of the anxiety and help them think clearly. If they know different ways to approach various types of questions they can feel better prepared. See the "Test-taking skills" section in the Appendix.

Chapter 12

Job Skills

Why are we talking about this?

Obtaining and maintaining employment can be difficult for anyone but it can be especially difficult for the individual with ASD. Since they have a hard time reading body language and tone of voice it can be difficult for them to understand what is expected of them in the work place. This chapter gives the teen the opportunity to talk about various situations that might arise in the work place.

Filling Out an Application: I Need a Job

Dante really wanted to get a car. He had gained his driver's license and his parents had put restrictions on how often he could take the family car. They told him if he got a job he could use the family car to get back and forth to work as long as they did not need the car. They also told him they would match whatever he saved toward a car.

Dante took the family car and picked up an application form at the local grocery store. A couple of his friends worked there and they told him the store was hiring. His friend's uncle was the manager so he thought getting the job would be easy. He had never filled out a job application before but he thought "How hard could it be?" He sat down and started filling it out in pen.

Dante had plans with his friends later that day so he wanted to get the application filled out as quickly as possible. He thought he could drop it off before he went out. While he was working on the application he messed up and put his first name where his last name should be. He scribbled it out and fixed it. He put in his school information, his grade point average, and when he was due to graduate. The next question asked if he had transportation to and from work. Since there were restrictions put on the car he wrote "maybe." Then it asked for previous job experience. Since this would be Dante's first job he put "none." Next it asked for any skills he might have that would make him a good candidate for the position. Dante was a personable young man and he found it easy to talk to people. Dante thought since he had never worked before it did not pertain to him so wrote "none." Finally it asked for the names, addresses, and phone numbers of three references. Dante wrote down names but did not write down contact information since he was unsure of their addresses. His parents asked him if he wanted them to look over the application before he dropped it off. He said no because he was in a hurry. He signed the application and dropped it back off at the grocery store.

A week went by and Dante had not been called for an interview. He decided to call his friend to see what was going on with the job. His friend told Dante they had hired someone earlier in the week. Dante was furious! He yelled at his friend and asked him why he did not put a good word in for him with his uncle? He knew Dante needed that job! His friend told him that he did talk to his uncle. His uncle said he could barely read the application and there were job responsibilities that involved writing down orders and stock. If he could not read the application how would others be able to read the orders? He just could not take the chance of hiring someone who could not take their time to write things down accurately so he hired someone else.

Discussion questions

- Since this was the first time Dante had filled out a job application should he have started filling it out in ink?

- What could he have done to avoid making mistakes and scribbling them out on the application?

- Should Dante have let his parents look over the application before he dropped it off?

- What could Dante have listed for qualifications that made him a good candidate for the job?

- What could Dante have done to prepare to give the information for the references?

What would you put in an application?

- Do you have all of your school information listed somewhere?

- What skills do you have that make you a good candidate for a job?

- What life experiences do you have that would pertain to the job you are applying for?

- Who would you list as references?

- Would you have someone look over the application before you turned it in?

Parent homework

The job application is the first impression an employer gets of your teen. Before they fill out an application have them make a "draft" application with all the necessary information. Then all they have to do is copy it from the "draft" to the final copy. Have them take their time and make sure it is legible. Go over the different skills your teen has so they know what to list. Make sure they have all the information for their references and that the people listed will give a good reference. Ask them if you could look over the final product to make sure everything is filled out correctly. Tell them it is OK to get more than one application for the same place just in case they make a mistake. Ask them to try to put themselves into the manager's position. If they saw the application they are turning in what would they think? If your teen cannot do that, you can play manager and go over it with them. Your teen will thank you when they get called for the interview.

Making a Good Impression: The Job Interview

Joel and Dayton both wanted to get a job at the mall working in their favorite clothing store Pumac. The store sold skater clothes, bikes, shoes, and skateboards. Both Joel and Dayton were excellent at extreme sports. This job would be perfect for either of them. They both filled out applications and dropped them off the same day. They were both very excited but the store was only able to hire one person.

The store manager Mr. Odesy called both Joel and Dayton to set up interviews. Dayton was very accommodating but Joel had an excuse for every time Mr. Odesy proposed. Finally Mr. Odesy asked Joel what day and time was good for him. Joel said he did not have any plans Thursday so the interview was set for Thursday at 9am.

Joel had his interview at 9am. He showed up ten minutes late for the interview. He was wearing a shirt that had stains on it, ripped dirty jeans, and had not showered in days so his hair was dirty and greasy. He had been working on his bike before the interview so there was grease all over his hands and under his nails. When he arrived at the interview Joel shook Mr. Odesy's hand and got him all greasy. When Mr. Odesy started asking questions Joel gave very short answers and acted like he did not care what Mr. Odesy was saying. At one point he told Mr. Odesy he sounded like he did not know anything about bikes and asked him how he became store manager in the first place. At the end of the interview he asked Joel if he had any questions and Joel replied "Are we done? I have things to do." Mr. Odesy said yes and Joel got up and left.

Dayton had his interview at 10am. He showed up 15 minutes early. He was wearing a nice button-down shirt, a good pair of dress pants, and he had had his hair cut the previous day. He greeted Mr. Odesy with a smile and a handshake. When Mr. Odesy started asking questions Dayton listened carefully and thought about his answers before he replied. Dayton even asked Mr. Odesy questions during the interview. He asked him how long the store had been in business, what types of sales goals they had for their employees, and if there was room for advancement with the company. Mr. Odesy was quite impressed with Dayton.

Neither Dayton or Joel had ever had a job before. The boys actually knew each other and rode together many times. They knew everything there was to know about the different types of bikes. They were both very informed when it came to the other merchandise in the store and both boys knew how to fix bikes quite well.

Discussion questions

- Who do you think the interviewer called to hire for the store? Why?
- What did Joel do wrong?
- What did Dayton do right?
- Do you think the "first impression" the interviewer got from each of the boys made a difference to whether or not they got hired?

What would you need to do to make your best impression if you were...

- Trying out for a school play?
- Explaining to the coach why you missed practice?
- Volunteering at a home for the elderly?
- Meeting the parents of your friend for the first time?
- Going on a job interview?

Parent homework

The next time you are out with your teen take the time to "people watch." Ask your teen what they think about people they see just by considering the way they look. Explain this is why the "first impression" is so important. Even though someone may have a wonderful personality you might not want to get to know them just because of their appearance. Explain that it may not be fair but people do make judgments so we should always try to look and act our best.

Dealing with Co-Workers: He Got the Promotion?!

Jules and Eli both worked at the Sell-Mart. They both got hired at the same time. They went through training together and Jules thought Eli would be a good employee. Some of the other trainees were talking negatively about Eli. They said he cheated on his training test. Jules did not see it happen so she did not judge either way.

One of the job requirements was to make up a goal sheet. Each employee needed to list the merchandise they would sell, how they would attempt to sell it, and set their own quota and deadline. Jules knew a lot about the exercise equipment so she used that on her goal sheet. Her goal involved selling exercise equipment by letting the customers try it before they buy it. This would involve having the equipment assembled and placed on the floor. She talked to Eli about her goal sheet and he thought it was a great idea. She asked him what his goal was and he said he had not thought about it yet. Jules suggested they work as a team on the same goal. That way they could double the sales. Eli agreed and said they could start next week. Jules told Eli she would train him on all the equipment.

The first thing that had to be done was to put together all of the equipment for the customers to try. Jules asked Eli if he could come in on Sunday to help her put together the equipment and set it up on the floor. He said he would meet her there. Eli did not show up at all. When Jules tried to call him she got his voicemail. She stayed until 9pm that evening getting everything set up.

When Eli came to work the next day he told Jules how great the display looked. All the machines were out and ready to go. Jules even put up fliers around the store and had the floor display set up like a gym with boxing ropes around it. Jules asked Eli where he was on Sunday and he said he had a family emergency but did not get into any detail. Jules said she would have liked at least a phone call. Eli apologized and said it would not happen again. Jules started training Eli on the equipment. He seemed to catch on quickly.

The manager approached Jules and Eli and complimented them on their display. Eli quickly thanked the manager and said it was his idea. He had told Jules how to set up the display to make it more attractive for customers. Jules was speechless! The manager patted Eli on the back and told him to keep up the good work. Then the manager turned to

Jules and told her she could learn a thing or two from Eli. Jules could not believe that Eli had taken credit for all of the work she had done.

They continued to work together to meet their sales goal. Jules would talk to customers and show them the correct way to use the equipment. She even suggested a healthy diet book that she had also displayed on the floor. The customers loved the individualized attention and sales were fantastic. While Jules was working with customers Eli would stand outside the ropes and talk to his friends. When the customers were ready he would check them out. He was no help to Jules at all. He did not even make one sale! Jules worked twice as hard to meet their quota and she did it! She was really proud of herself but she would never work with Eli on a project again.

It came time for their performance reviews. The manager called Eli in first for his review. Eli came out of the manager's office smiling and told Jules he had just been given a raise and had been promoted to the exercise equipment supervisor. Jules thought that if Eli had been promoted to supervisor for all the work she had done then she must be getting a manager's position. She went into the evaluation excited to hear what was in store for her.

When she walked in the manager asked her to sit down. He told her that Eli had explained how they put together the goal and worked on meeting it. He was very proud of Eli for meeting the sales goal and told Jules she should work harder next time. Jules tried to explain to the manager that she had done all of the sales. The manager told her that all the checkout receipts had Eli's employee number on them so he got credit for all the sales. Unfortunately, due to the amount of sales Eli had made the corporate office gave the decision to give him the promotion. Jules' manager told her to hang in there. Jules told her manager she quit and stormed out of the office.

Discussion questions

- Was it a good idea for Jules to work with Eli on the goal sheet? Why or why not?

- What should Jules have done when Eli did not show up to help her set up all the equipment?

- What should Jules have done when Eli took credit for the display?

- Do you think Jules should have quit her job? What other options did she have?

- What would you have done if you were Jules and someone took credit for your work?

What would you do with a co-worker in these situations?

- Your co-worker is the manager's son and stands around all day. You have to do twice the work.

- You ask your co-worker to do something for you and they do not do it. You get into trouble because the job is not done.

- Your co-worker starts a rumor about you at work.

- Your co-worker messes up and blames you.

- Your co-worker calls you ten minutes before the shift starts and asks you if you could cover for them. You say no and they tell the boss they asked you last week and you said you would do it but you changed your mind.

Parent homework

Sometimes co-workers can be quite difficult to deal with. For some reason there is always that one person who does not do what they are supposed to do. Talk to your teen about their job. If there is someone there causing them aggravation they will probably mention it to you. Talk to them about how to deal with difficult co-workers. Each situation will be different. Help them list their options. Sometimes there may not be an easy solution. Then talk to your teen about whether or not the position is worth the amount of stress it may be causing them. Make a "pro" versus a "con" list. If they love their job but one person is making it difficult help them reframe their thoughts. If they are not fond of their job to begin with and someone is making it more difficult for them help them decide if it is worth it to stay or if they should start looking for a different position.

Dealing with a Difficult Boss: The Boss Has No Clue!

Jennsen was a senior and she had had the same job since she was a sophomore in high school. She loved her job. When she first started working at the store she was only working for the summer but she did such a great job the supervisor asked her if she wanted to continue to work part-time while she was in school. Jennsen knew everything there was to know about the store. She could not advance into a supervisory position because she was unable to work full time while she was in school. Everyone went to her with their questions.

The supervisor had resigned from his position to take a position with a different store. The store hired Ms. Hayden to take his place. When Ms. Hayden started the store manager asked Jennsen to show her around and explain the policies and procedures to her. Jennsen had received fantastic reviews from her previous supervisor and the manager knew she was the perfect person to show Ms. Hayden how the store ran. Jennsen felt honored to have been asked and was excited to show Ms. Hayden around.

Jennsen met Ms. Hayden in the manager's office the next day. Ms. Hayden seemed very nice and said she was happy to be working so closely with Jennsen. As soon as they walked out of the office Ms. Hayden's personality changed. She told Jennsen that she had been in the store business for over 15 years and she did not think that Jennsen was qualified to tell her how to do her job. She told Jennsen to get to work and walked away.

Jennsen was shocked by Ms. Hayden's words but she did as she was told. A few weeks later the store started falling apart. Inventory was lost, employees were getting upset, and it seemed every time anyone went to Ms. Hayden for help she had no idea what they were talking about. Everyone started going to Jennsen for help. Jennsen started straightening up all the issues with the store. Jennsen would have helped everyone anyway but her employee review was coming up and she thought this would look good to the store manager.

When Ms. Hayden found out Jennsen was fixing the issues she started giving Jennsen other assignments in the store to keep her busy so she did not have time to help everyone else. Jennsen thought the assignments were ridiculous. Every day Jennsen came into the store she was assigned to check the inventory. After she got done Ms. Hayden would tell her to check it again. Jennsen was always doing everything twice! Every time she turned around Ms. Hayden was there. When anyone else needed Ms. Hayden for something she was nowhere to be found. Jennsen felt she was being singled out because Ms. Hayden did not like her.

When Jennsen received her employee review she was appalled. On a scale of one to five, one being the lowest and five being the highest, Ms. Hayden had given Jennsen all ones! Jennsen had always received fours and fives on her review. When she asked Ms. Hayden why she had received such a poor review Ms. Hayden did not respond.

Discussion questions

- Do you think the store manager should have asked Jennsen to show Ms. Hayden around?

- Do you think Ms. Hayden should have taken the time with Jennsen to learn the policies and procedures of the store?

- Why do you think Ms. Hayden did not want to listen to Jennsen?

- Why do you think Ms. Hayden gave Jennsen a bad review?

- What do you think Jennsen should have done when she received the bad review?

How would you handle this situation with your boss?

- Your boss asks you to do something you know has already been done.

- Your boss loses your time off request sheet.

- Your boss tells you that you are required to work overtime on the weekend that you are supposed to be going away with your family.

- Your boss tells you to do something you know is incorrect.

- Your boss makes inappropriate comments to you while you are at work.

Parent homework

Unfortunately most of us have had a boss at one time or another who had absolutely no clue what was involved with our position. It is especially difficult when you love your job and someone comes in and then you hate to even go to work. Usually the problem takes care of itself over time and that boss winds up leaving but occasionally this does not happen. Talk to your teen if they have a boss that is just a bit too much to take. Ask them what they like about their position. Ask them if they think it is worth it to stay or if they think they should leave. Talk to them about the financial issues they may encounter if they leave their current position without first finding another one. If your teen's boss is inappropriate with your teen, talk to them about the options they may have. Going above your immediate boss's head and explaining the problem to upper management may help solve the issues. Tell your teen to be prepared if upper management does not want to listen. Role play different situations with your teen. Hopefully it will work out for the best no matter what happens. If not, they can always find another position that they might like even more.

Advancement: This Could Be a Career

Kara was a junior in high school and had had many different jobs throughout her high school career. She had worked in various retail stores and fast food restaurants. This was the first time she had received a position in an office and she loved it! She was hired as the part-time evening and weekend administrative assistant to the manager of a local company. Every day after school she would go to the company and take over from the full-time day administrative assistant. She would have different assignments for Kara to complete every day. During the week Kara was responsible for typing memos, emailing them to the appropriate departments, filing, answering phones, and taking messages. On the weekends she also greeted customers and helped with their orders. Dealing with the customers was her favorite part of the job.

Kara knew she could not work full time due to school but she really enjoyed working for this company. She thought she would like to continue to work there after graduation. Maybe she would be able to get into sales since she enjoyed working with the customers so much.

Kara decided to talk to the manager. When she went into his office to talk to him about advancement he asked her if she would like to work full time in the summer. She happily said yes. Then he told her to talk with the personnel office to find out if advancement could be an option.

Personnel told her she would need a business degree to get into the sales department full time. Kara went into school and talked with her guidance counselor. She wanted to find out what she needed to do to get into a college to get the business degree. Kara's guidance counselor told her about local colleges that offered the program and said she might be able to start as soon as the summer. The college was offering programs to students who were going into their senior year and she would be able to get college credits. Kara did not know what to do. If she went to school in the summer she would not be able to work full time in the office. Kara decided to think about her options.

Discussion questions

- Do you think sales would be a good job for Kara? Why?
- Do you think Kara's manager thought she was good at her job? Why?
- Do you think Kara should work full time in the summer or work part time and take the college classes?
- Do you think it would jeopardize Kara's job if she took the college classes and only worked part time?
- What would you do if you were Kara?

Would these things help you advance in your career?

- Learning different aspects of the company you work for.
- Applying for different positions in the company.
- Taking company trainings.
- Taking college classes.
- Talking to your supervisor/manager.

Parent homework

It is wonderful if your teen finds something while they are young that they want to turn into a career. Guide your teen through ways to advance. Have them take courses and/or trainings offered even if they are not of interest to them. It will help them see the bigger picture of what is going on with the company. Talk to them about having a good relationship with their management and the other employees. People skills are very important if you want to advance in your career. Tell them to talk to the personnel department or management and ask questions about different advancement opportunities with the company. Who knows, maybe your teen will be the next CEO of the company.

Appendix

Ways to reduce stress

Count to ten
Write a story
Walk away
Play an instrument
Think about something that
makes you happy
Write in a journal
Think of a relaxing place
Play cards
Ride your scooter, bike,
skateboard, etc.
Kick something
Dance around
Scream and stomp
Go for a walk, run, jog, etc.
Punch a pillow
Scream into a pillow
Talk to a friend
Clean
Jump on a trampoline
Find a quiet spot
Squeeze a stuffed animal
Squeeze a stress ball
Talk to your pet
Beat up your stuffed animals
Talk about how your body is
feeling
Play a video game
Talk on the phone
Listen to music
Call your doctor
Watch TV
Read a book
Go on a swing
Smile and laugh
Play on the computer
Chew gum
Take a nap
Play with toys
Go swimming
Talk about it
Take a shower
Have a snack
Draw
Break sticks and throw them at
trees
Lie down
Throw rocks into the water
Play with friends or family
Go fishing

Climb a tree

Exercise

Play outside

Play sports

Write poems

Do some slow breathing

Lie in the sun

Go shopping

Watch birds

Bounce on a ball

Go to the beach

Play a board game

Watch fish

Paint

Play with pets

Meditate

Have a friendly wrestle

Go horseback riding

Build something

Go for a drive

Test-taking skills

How to reduce anxiety before a test

- Ask the teacher what may be on the upcoming test. (Note: if the teacher gave you notes that is probably what will be on the test.)

- Do not cram for the test; study throughout the week before the test.

- Create your own test with the material that will be covered and quiz yourself.

- Get a good night's sleep before the day of the test.

- Eat breakfast.

- Wear comfortable clothes.

- Write your name on the test.

- Take a couple of deep breaths and let them out slowly before you begin the test.

- Count to ten.

- Read the directions carefully; if you are not sure about something ask the teacher.

Throughout the test

- If time permits read over the entire test before beginning.
- Make notes on the test of things you remember.
- Answer the questions you know first.
- Try not to leave anything blank; it is better to guess and possibly get partial credit than to leave it blank and not get any credit for the question at all.
- If time permits, review your answers.
- Remember, your teacher does not want you to fail so if you are unsure about a question ask for help.
- Do not stress if other students have finished before you.
- After you hand the test in do not stress about it.

Multiple choice questions

- Read the question carefully.
- Circle, underline, or highlight important words in the question.
- Eliminate the answers you know are incorrect.
- Look over the remaining choices carefully before choosing your answer.
- Look over other portions of the test to see if there are hints for the answer.
- If you are not sure, take a guess.
- If one of the choices is "All of the above" and you know that two or more choices are correct then "All of the above" is probably the correct answer.

"True or False" questions

- Read the question carefully.
- Circle, underline, or highlight important information in the question.

- Look for key words such as "always," "never," "every."
- If a statement contains two negative words or prefixes cross out both because two negatives usually make a positive.
- If any part of the question is false the answer is false.
- If part of the question is true that does not make the answer true.
- If you are not sure take a guess.

Essay questions

- Read the question carefully.
- Make sure you understand what the question is asking you to do.
- If you are unsure of what to do ask the teacher.
- Do an outline first using key words, and perhaps use a graphic organizer (a visual aid that is used to help people organize their thoughts).
- Take your time and write neatly so your teacher can read your answer.
- If you feel you may need additional time to complete the essay talk to your teacher.
- Try to use an introduction, body, and conclusion in your answer.

Short answer questions

- Read the directions carefully.
- Circle, underline, or highlight key words in the question.
- Immediately write down what you remember somewhere on the test.
- Do not leave an answer blank; if you are not sure write down your thoughts, you might get partial credit.
- If you think there may be more than one correct answer ask the teacher what you should do.

- If the question has multiple parts make sure you have answered all of them.

Open book tests

- Do not think you do not have to study for an open book test.
- Read over the chapter(s) that are going to be included so you have a general idea where the information is.
- Use highlighting tape to mark key words in paragraphs.
- Place bookmarks with topics listed in the pages with important information.
- Bring everything the teacher allows you to bring: book, notebook, etc.
- Read the question carefully.
- List page numbers where you found your answer.
- Try to put the answer in your own words instead of copying the information exactly as it is written in the book.

Math tests

- Create your own quiz and do practice problems before the test.
- Ask your teacher if you can use a formula sheet, calculator, or other resource if needed.
- If you are unable to use a formula sheet, write the formulas down somewhere on the test as soon as you receive it.
- Read the question carefully. (Are you seeing a pattern here?)
- Group the problems and do all the same type of problem at the same time (all addition, subtraction, etc.).
- Make sure you show all your work.
- Even if you think your answer is wrong do not erase the work; you may get partial credit.

Oral tests

- Make sure you have a list of the topics that may be presented.

- Study all the topics carefully.

- Practice giving your answer in front of family, friends, or a mirror, or video-tape yourself.

- If you are allowed to use resources make sure they are clearly marked (use bookmarks in books, bookmark pages online, highlight notes, prepare note cards, etc.).

- If you are allowed to use a computer as a resource make sure it works before you present.

- Be early for the test.

- Listen carefully to the topic the teacher gives you.

- If you are unsure about the question, ask for clarification.

- Keep eye contact and proper posture.

- Avoid being monotone and use inflection in your voice.

- Try to pace your speaking so you do not speak too fast or too slow.

- Answer in complete sentences and try to avoid overusing nervous words such as "like" or "um."

- Answer any questions asked with more than a "yes" or "no"; give detail.

- When you are done thank your audience for their time and attention.